SYMPOSIA OF THE SECTION ON MICROBIOLOGY
THE NEW YORK ACADEMY OF MEDICINE

Number 1
DIAGNOSIS OF VIRAL AND
RICKETTSIAL INFECTIONS

DIAGNOSIS OF VIRAL AND RICKETTSIAL INFECTIONS

EDITED BY

Frank L. Horsfall, Jr.

SYMPOSIUM HELD AT THE
NEW YORK ACADEMY OF MEDICINE
JANUARY 29 AND 30, 1948

1949   New York
COLUMBIA UNIVERSITY PRESS

COPYRIGHT 1949 NEW YORK
COLUMBIA UNIVERSITY PRESS

PUBLISHED IN GREAT BRITAIN
AND INDIA
BY GEOFFREY CUMBERLEGE
OXFORD UNIVERSITY PRESS
LONDON AND BOMBAY

MANUFACTURED IN THE UNITED STATES OF AMERICA

SECTION ON MICROBIOLOGY
THE NEW YORK ACADEMY OF MEDICINE

Officers
GREGORY SHWARTZMAN, *Chairman*
HARRY MOST, *Secretary*

Advisory Board
JOHN G. KIDD
RENÉ J. DUBOS
FRANK L. HORSFALL, JR.
COLIN M. MACLEOD
RALPH S. MUCKENFUSS

Organizing Committee for Symposium No. 1
FRANK L. HORSFALL, JR., *Chairman*
RALPH S. MUCKENFUSS
GREGORY SHWARTZMAN

Foreword

ON MAY 1, 1947, the Fellowship of The New York Academy of Medicine approved the organization of the Section on Microbiology, thus establishing the first section of the Academy devoted to basic medical sciences.

Ample opportunities are already available for presentation and publication of scientific papers. However, with increasing diversity, complexity, and specialization, there is evident a need for opportunity to digest and correlate the rapidly accumulating body of new knowledge. The main objectives of the new Section are to provide a forum for the exchange of information amongst the workers engaged in basic and clinical sciences.

Accordingly, the scope of interest of the Section on Microbiology is broadly defined, as embodying the following: (1) bacteriology, mycology and parasitology; (2) viruses and rickettsiae; (3) maladies of unknown or uncertain etiology, possibly of infectious origin; (4) immunology; (5) chemotherapy; (6) pathology relative to microbiology; and (7) methods of study adopted from related sciences, as applied to microbiology. The programs of meetings of the Section are arranged to deal with single topics in their various aspects. In addition to regular monthly evening meetings, several symposia are organized yearly, each consisting of consecutive afternoon and evening sessions. The participants present extensive reviews in their particular fields of endeavor, thus bringing correlated and authoritative scientific data and concepts to the attention of the microbiologists and allied laboratory and clinical investigators. Unpublished symposia are soon forgotten, but their benefits may be retained by prompt publication. Important service is rendered by the Columbia University Press which has undertaken the publication of this series under the auspices of the New York Academy of Medicine and the editorship of the respective chairmen of the symposia.

GREGORY SHWARTZMAN

Contents

    FOREWORD   ix
    GREGORY SHWARTZMAN

1. INTRODUCTION   3
   FRANK L. HORSFALL, JR., *Hospital of The Rockefeller Institute for Medical Research*

2. LABORATORY DIAGNOSTIC PROCEDURES FOR INFLUENZA   5
   GEORGE K. HIRST, *Division of Infectious Diseases, The Public Health Research Institute of The City of New York, Inc.*

3. THE DIAGNOSIS OF MUMPS   15
   GERTRUDE HENLE AND WERNER HENLE, *The Children's Hospital of Philadelphia, Department of Pediatrics, School of Medicine, University of Pennsylvania*

4. THE DIAGNOSIS OF INFECTIONS CAUSED BY THE PSITTACOSIS-LYMPHOGRANULOMA GROUP OF VIRUSES, INCLUDING TRACHOMA AND INCLUSION BLENNORRHEA   25
   GEOFFREY RAKE, *The Squibb Institute for Medical Research*

5. THE DIAGNOSIS OF PRIMARY ATYPICAL PNEUMONIA   42
   FRANK L. HORSFALL, JR., *Hospital of The Rockefeller Institute for Medical Research*

6. THE DIAGNOSIS OF NEUROTROPIC VIRUS INFECTIONS, INCLUDING THE VIRAL ENCEPHALITIDES, LYMPHOCYTIC CHORIOMENINGITIS, AND POLIOMYELITIS   57
   JORDI CASALS AND PETER K. OLITSKY, *The Rockefeller Institute for Medical Research*

7. THE DIAGNOSIS OF INFECTION WITH THE VIRUS OF HERPES SIMPLEX   83
   T. F. MCNAIR SCOTT, LEWIS L. CORIELL, AND HARVEY

BLANK, *The Children's Hospital of Philadelphia, Department of Pediatrics and Department of Dermatology and Syphilology, School of Medicine, University of Pennsylvania*

8. THE DIAGNOSIS OF RABIES 92
HARALD N. JOHNSON, *The International Health Division, The Rockefeller Foundation*

9. THE DIAGNOSIS OF DENGUE 101
R. WALTER SCHLESINGER, *Division of Infectious Diseases, The Public Health Research Institute of The City of New York, Inc.*

10. THE DIAGNOSIS OF INFECTIOUS MONONUCLEOSIS 108
JOHN R. PAUL, *Section of Preventive Medicine, Yale University School of Medicine*

11. THE DIAGNOSIS OF EPIDEMIC, MURINE, AND SCRUB TYPHUS, AS WELL AS Q FEVER 117
JOSEPH E. SMADEL, *Department of Virus and Rickettsial Diseases, Army Medical Department Research and Graduate School, Army Medical Center*

12. THE DIAGNOSIS OF ROCKY MOUNTAIN SPOTTED FEVER AND RICKETTSIALPOX 133
HERALD R. COX, *Section of Viral and Rickettsial Research, Lederle Laboratories Division, American Cyanamid Company*

13. THE DIAGNOSIS OF INFECTIOUS HEPATITIS 147
W. PAUL HAVENS, JR., *The Jefferson Medical College*

DIAGNOSIS OF VIRAL AND RICKETTSIAL INFECTIONS

Chapter 1

INTRODUCTION

By Frank L. Horsfall, Jr., *Hospital of The Rockefeller Institute for Medical Research*

As a result of the critical studies of numerous investigators during recent years, the diagnosis of many viral and rickettsial infections has been placed on a secure footing. By means of extremely sensitive and highly specific reactions it is now possible to determine the presence and establish the identity of a number of the smallest of known infectious agents. Similarly, some of the subtle alterations in immunological status which result from infections with certain viruses or rickettsiae can be detected and measured with a degree of precision.

A number of the workers who have been responsible, in large measure, for recent developments in this field have been kind enough to participate in the present symposium. They have graciously undertaken the labor of discussing present information as concerns the diagnosis of each of a total of at least thirty-two specific infectious diseases caused either by viruses or by rickettsiae.

The principles which form the basis for the accurate diagnosis of infections induced by viral or rickettsial agents are in no way different from those long-since established with infections of other sorts. Recovery and identification of the infectious agent is the first objective. Evidence regarding the causal relationship of the agent to the infectious process is the second. Because of the peculiar properties of viruses and rickettsiae, the technical procedures necessary for the achievement of either objective are more or less elaborate. As a consequence, they may require unusual facilities, considerable skill, and much time.

The recovery of either a virus or a rickettsia necessitates the use of a susceptible living host or tissue, and, as a consequence, it is highly impracticable to attempt the direct recovery of such agents from more than a relatively small number of cases. In general, it is somewhat less difficult to obtain indirect evidence from which the nature and identity of the agent responsible for the infection may be deduced. Whenever possible, serological procedures are employed in order that the development of antibodies specifically directed against the agent may be demonstrated. *In vitro* techniques, as, for example, complement fixation and hemagglutination inhibition, possess obvious advantages over *in vivo* procedures, such as neutralization tests which require the use of experimental animals, but involve a certain risk relative to specificity and require careful control.

In certain infections, procedures suitable for the recovery of the etiological agent and the demonstration of the development of antibodies against it are not yet available. In such instances, as an example, in infectious hepatitis, important information has been acquired by employing human volunteers in transmission experiments. In other instances, for example, in infectious mononucleosis or in primary atypical pneumonia, the occurrence of unusual serological phenomena may provide the basis for useful laboratory procedures, which are of great aid in diagnosis.

Although throughout the symposium major emphasis will be placed on a critical evaluation of laboratory procedures which are helpful in establishing a diagnosis, it should be pointed out that available techniques provide no simple or ready means for making an accurate diagnosis and do not diminish the importance of carefully obtained clinical findings. Many present procedures have definite limitations, and these will be emphasized.

In each of the sessions the diagnosis of at least one disease about which much more information is needed will be discussed, and the deficiencies in present knowledge will be clearly evident. A number of viral infections, in particular the common exanthemata of childhood, are not included because there are no satisfactory laboratory procedures which are useful in establishing the diagnosis.

Chapter 2

LABORATORY DIAGNOSTIC PROCEDURES
FOR INFLUENZA

By GEORGE K. HIRST, *Division of Infectious Diseases, The Public Health Research Institute of The City of New York, Inc.*

For the discussion of laboratory diagnosis, influenza may be defined as a respiratory disease which occurs characteristically in epidemic form and is caused by two antigenically distinct types of virus known as influenza A and B. These two virus types cause very similar disease pictures but differ in their epidemiological behavior. In the United States, influenza A epidemics have occurred at intervals of two and three years, while influenza B outbreaks have so far occurred at intervals of four and six years. Many small, localized outbreaks may precede a major wave, which then sweeps the country in two to four months' time. The incidence in the total population may be even 20 percent or higher. Since 1933 all major outbreaks have been due to either influenza A or influenza B, and there is no necessity at the present time to postulate further virus types to explain the epidemic disease. Between epidemic periods, influenza-like cases occur sporadically, but only a small percentage can be shown to have infection with influenza A or B virus. The great majority are of unknown etiology.

In influenza the causative agent is present in the secretions of the upper respiratory tract during the acute phase of the illness, and infection is followed by a rise in specific virus antibody level in the circulating blood. These two phenomena are the bases for the methods of laboratory diagnosis. In addition to the numerous cases of clinical influenza during an epidemic there are numerous cases of inapparent infection, usually in much higher incidence than the clinical disease, and this is a fact which greatly influences the behavior of epidemics as well as the interpretation of laboratory data.

While there are two antigenic types of influenza virus, there are substrains within each of these categories. In some cases they are only distantly related to each other, a circumstance that greatly increases the difficulty of laboratory diagnosis, especially in type identification. The behavior of strains on primary isolation in chick embryos is also quite variable from epidemic to epidemic, which makes it difficult to lay down rigid rules for virus isolation or to predict accurately the efficacy of a given method in a new epidemic.

The laboratory diagnosis of influenza has been possible only during the past fifteen years, and since then the methods employed have undergone radical changes. There is nothing to suggest that today's technique will not undergo further changes such as have occurred with the problems brought by each succeeding epidemic. The two main methods of laboratory diagnosis are the isolation of virus from throat washings and the comparison of serological antibody levels at the acute and convalescent stages of infection. While other methods have been used in the past, such as the inoculation of ferrets for virus isolation or the performance of neutralization tests in mice, it is now generally agreed that the diagnosis can be made most simply either by purely *in vitro* serological techniques or by the inoculation of chick embryos with throat washings.

Of the two methods to be discussed, virus isolation and antibody titration, the former has certain advantages in that the result is obtained faster and, when positive, is usually unequivocal. The disadvantages of the isolation method are almost entirely technical, but are of such a nature that they may be easily overcome. Human influenza virus can be isolated in chick embryos by either allantoic or amniotic inoculation. While the allantoic method is extremely simple the amiotic technique is superior in results.

Throat washings should be selected, if there is a choice, from those patients who are most recently and most acutely ill. There is a diminishing possibility of recovering virus after the onset, and the chances are negligible after five or six days. Water, broth, saline, or a buffer solution may be used for a gargle, with or without the addition of inactivated horse serum. It is advisable to include some penicillin in the washing, as much as 500 units per c.c., to inhibit the growth of organisms from the throat. The patient is asked to cough before gargling in order to bring up possibly infective material from the trachea and bronchi.

The best results are obtained when eggs are inoculated shortly after the washing is obtained; if the delay is more than a few hours the material should be frozen, preferably at a low temperature. By far the best results are obtained on inoculating embryos of thirteen days' incubation, though this may vary slightly depending on the incubator temperature. Younger embryos frequently give negative results with material which is clearly positive in embryos of thirteen days. The reason for this difference may be that the inoculated virus does not get to the lung until swallowing and respiratory movements of the embryo begin.

Any method of amniotic inoculation is satisfactory as long as it is certain that the material gets into the proper place. Taylor and Chialvo (1) have worked out a method of inoculating through the air sac, which has the advantage of avoiding the hemorrhage which occurs on dropping the membrane. The method which we are currently using is essentially the same as that described by Beveridge and Burnet (2). It consists in cutting a window, dropping the chorioallantoic membrane, pulling the amniotic sac out through a hole in the allantoic sac, and inoculating under direct vision. The throat washing should contain enough penicillin so that each embryo will receive 200 to 400 units. This is an excess, but is desirable in that it reduces the mortality from bacterial infection to the lowest possible figure. After inoculation the eggs should be incubated at 35°C. They may be examined after two or three days, but optimal results are not obtained until the fourth and sometimes the fifth day. When the eggs are opened, the allantoic fluid is poured off and the amniotic fluid is aspirated with a wide-mouthed pipette. The yield of amniotic fluid is small, averaging less than 1 c.c., and some sacs are dry and have to be washed out with saline. The fluids are harvested separately and tested individually for hemagglutinin titer by the pattern method. Both fowl and guinea pig red cells should be used for testing. The former give the fewest false positive reactions, while the guinea pig cell agglutinins are sometimes present in much higher titer than those for fowl cells. A good positive fluid should give agglutination in a final dilution of 1:500 or higher, and titers in the neighborhood of 1:16 or less should be regarded with suspicion, since normal amniotic fluid, especially with guinea pig cells, gives very deceptive reactions in this range. It is a good rule to regard any doubtful test as negative pending further passage by either the amniotic or the allantoic route. With most strains the allantoic route is adequate for secondary passage, but with the strains of 1947, adaptation to the allantoic sac was very slow and difficult.

The occurrence of high titer agglutinins in amniotic fluids is good presumptive evidence of the presence of influenza virus, but the agent in such fluids should always be typed. This is sometimes much more easily said than done, because newly isolated strains are inhibited in agglutination to an unusual degree by normal sera, and in 1947 the influenza A strains were almost impossible to type by ordinary methods, that is, demonstration of specific agglutination inhibition by influenza A immune sera. This difficulty was enhanced by the very small degree of cross relationship between these strains and the usual types maintained in the laboratory. Such difficulties in strain typing can be overcome in part by: (a) using immune antisera of very high antibody content; (b) using sera made with strains closely allied to those being typed; (c) the repeated passage of a strain in the allantoic sac which will lower the extent of inhibition caused by normal sera; (d) employing convalescent influenza A and B human sera, a method which is sometimes successful when immune sera of other species fail; (e) typing strains by complement fixation; and finally (f) exhausting typing sera of their content of normal inhibitor by means of sodium periodate or culture filtrates of cholera vibrio. While the technique for the use of these agents has not been fully worked out, preliminary results suggest that they may be useful and lead to a solution of this difficult problem.

Having isolated, cultivated, and typed a strain of influenza virus, we have obtained almost unequivocal evidence of influenzal infection, and this is laboratory diagnosis in its quickest and most definitive form. The only reservation which needs to be applied to the interpretation of a successful isolation is the possibility of laboratory contamination. This possibility must not be taken lightly, especially in a laboratory where *in vitro* tests with active virus are being carried out. The chances of contamination are greatest when the isolation is achieved by repeated passage of material in embryos and the passage material is exposed to room air for a time.

While influenza virus may be isolated in other ways (for example, in ferrets, hamsters, or mice), none of these methods are equal to the amniotic inoculation of embryos in speed, sensitivity in virus detection, or convenience. The only method of comparable value is the allantoic inoculation of chick embryos; this has simplicity as its main virtue, since it can be performed by individuals with little or no prior experience with chick embryos. In some outbreaks this method has given very creditable results, but in the last two epidemics (1945-46 and 1947) it failed almost completely. In comparative experiments with throat washings which contained large amounts of virus, the allantoic route required 10,000 times as much inoculum as the amniotic route for a positive result. The former cannot be recommended for routine use.

The ease with which influenza virus may be isolated by the amniotic method varies enormously in different years. In some epidemics 60 to 70 percent of the serologically proven cases tested had positive throat washings, while in other outbreaks the figure has dropped to as low as 25 percent. It is obvious that a negative result does not rule out influenza, and, in order to establish a diagnosis in an epidemic, a selection of six or more washings from the best cases, inoculated into six or more eggs each, is the best guarantee of successful diagnosis in a short time.

The other method of laboratory diagnosis is the measurement of a rise in antibody titer during convalescence by means of complement-fixation or agglutination-inhibition tests. While this method gives diagnosis in retrospect only, it is important because it can be performed by laboratories without facilities for eggs and requires only routine bacteriological equipment. As with most other virus diseases, it is imperative to compare two sera, and this is especially true of influenza, since all adults possess circulating antibody. As can be seen in a comparison of normal and convalescent phase levels in a large population, there is considerable overlapping, so that even the possession of a high level of antibodies in an individual is not certain evidence of convalescence from influenza. A diagnosis is possible on the basis of a comparison between sera taken as late as the sixth day of the disease and as soon as ten days after onset, though a larger interval is more desirable.

The detection of a rise in antibody titer by complement fixation with allantoic fluid antigens is very successful; the magnitude of the antibody rise is of the same order as that obtained with agglutination-inhibition tests, and there is no difficulty with a normal inhibitor. In recent years the agglutination-inhibition test has been the most widely employed of *in vitro* techniques. The most useful form of this test for general use is known as the pattern test, the details of which have been fully described by Salk (3) and which is recommended by the following advantages: (a) ease of performance; (b) sharp, easily interpreted, end points; (c) lack of need for special equipment; (d) wide variation in incubation time before reading which is permissible; (e) economy of materials, virus, and serum.

The materials required for the test are virus strains, types A and B, prepared from allantoic fluid, and red cells. These may be either avian cells obtained from a slaughterhouse, guinea pig cells, human group O cells, or sheep cells as used in the modification of the method recently described by Magill and Sugg (4). The virus may be prepared long ahead of time, keeps well at refrigerator temperatures, and, without doubt, if the demand is sufficient, may be obtained from commercial sources. A constant amount of virus (about four agglutinating units) is added to falling twofold dilutions of serum. The amount of virus may be varied over a wide range without affecting the test adversely. After serum and virus are mixed, red cells in 1 to ¼ percent concentration are added, and the test is allowed to stand at room temperature for 1 to 1½ hours. In tubes without agglutination the cells settle in a sharply outlined small button, while with agglutination the cells settle in a diffuse disc on the bottom of the tube, frequently with a characteristically serrated edge. The end points are quite easy to read; usually not more than one tube is equivocal. By this method the demonstration of fourfold or greater differences in antibody titer between simultaneously tested serum pairs is significant of influenza infection. Because of inherent inaccuracies in the method it is not felt that twofold rises can be relied on as surely significant, and this is the main drawback of the method. As with virus isolation, the percentage of positive serological results obtained in typical clinical cases varies with the epidemic, the type of strain involved, and the preepidemic antibody level of the population, but an average figure would probably be 60 to 75 percent of the cases tested.

Another antibody titration method (5) employs a photoelectric densitometer for measurement of the agglutination. This method has the advantage that twofold differences of antibody level are a significant indication of infection, so that in a given series of sera more positive diagnoses can be returned than with the pattern method.

This technique consumes much more time and materials in performance and requires a densitometer as special equipment. Nevertheless, there is no doubt that it is a superior method of antibody measurement, more objective, more precise and quantitative than the pattern method; but whether or not it is used depends on the level of precision required.

Human infection with influenza virus may result in an antibody response which ranges from no detectable change to a 100-fold or greater increase in circulating antibody level. In an influenza epidemic there are usually more silent or inapparent infections than clinically manifest ones, and there is no difference in mean antibody response between these two groups. The strain specificity of the human response is incompletely understood, but often greater increases in antibody titer are detected by testing with strains from the epidemic than by the use of distantly related ones. In interpreting the results of serological tests it is well to keep these facts in mind. It is obvious that a negative test does not rule out infection, even when the sera have been tested with many strains and by a technique with which a two-fold rise is significant. It is also possible that an antibody rise does not necessarily mean that the illness in question was influenza, since it may reflect the result of silent infection, the illness having been due to some other agent. Besides these reservations and the possibility that the individual has been recently vaccinated with influenza virus, there are no qualifications which need to be placed on a serological diagnosis in which there is a rise of a magnitude deemed significant for the technique used. No false positive increases in influenza antibodies have been reported. However, the finding of a very high titer in a single convalescent serum specimen is of no diagnostic value, since the range in variation of titers in a normal population is enormous.

When one is called on to establish the etiology of a respiratory epidemic, it is almost always the case that the outbreak has been present for some time and was not noticed or taken seriously until the cases became numerous. In such instances it is possible to make a definite diagnosis in a few hours and under field conditions. Of the wide variety of antibody levels in a population, influenza tends to pick out those possessing less than average antibody titer for the agent in question. By bleeding eight or ten acutely ill cases and an equal number of convalescents and titering their sera, either individually or in pools, with A and B virus it can readily be decided whether or not influenza is involved and what type. If the inciting agent is influenza type A, the convalescent cases may have a geometric mean titer four or more times greater than that of the acutely ill, while the mean B levels should show no significant difference. This sort of test can be done in the field with little equipment. Where used so far it has given information which agreed with later studies of virus isolation, and it should be more widely used.

There are two main ways of making a laboratory diagnosis of influenza: virus isolation, and the establishment of a significant rise in antibody titer on convalescence. Both methods have their shortcomings and both are so new as to be fairly certain of further refinement. Even in combination, both methods frequently fail to make a positive diagnosis in all cases, but they are at present the only workable ways of making a certain diagnosis.

It may be profitable briefly to review the need for laboratory methods from the standpoint of the routine bacteriological laboratory, that is, a laboratory serving a hospital or the practicing physician. There are two main problems, the sporadic and the epidemic case. The sporadic illness with typical influenzal symptoms is so rarely caused by influenza viruses, either A or B, that the application of diagnostic methods to such cases becomes tedious and unrewarding. Furthermore, a knowledge of the etiology in a rare sporadic case does not materially alter the conduct of treatment, especially since the information comes late in the disease. It cannot be expected that the private practitioner will take much interest in these diagnostic procedures, and certainly very few cases are admitted to hospitals. At the present time, most requests for a diagnosis of influenza in private practice concern cases in which the question of influenza has arisen only after all other possibilities have been exhausted, at a time so late in the disease that it is no longer possible to make a laboratory diagnosis.

The investigation of the etiology of epidemic outbreaks is another matter, and the facilities for doing this should be widely available, since it is the only method of arriving at a definite conclusion concerning the nature of an outbreak. In the event of an epidemic, however, it is usually not possible, nor highly desirable, to make a laboratory diagnosis in every case; the main function of a laboratory is to establish without question the nature of the etiology in a small number of typical cases. On the basis of positive results the physicians of a community will usually, with considerable justification, diagnose all febrile respiratory illnesses of a minor nature as influenza. In fact, a laboratory diagnosis of influenza A made in a New York City epidemic may be said to have a considerable degree of validity when applied to an outbreak in Cleveland, for example, if it is clear, as is often the case, that both epidemics are part of the same major episode.

The limitations described above for the usefulness of laboratory diagnosis of influenza apply only to its use as a routine test for diagnosis in the sense of the Wassermann reaction; it is not intended in any way to discourage the widespread use of these methods for bacteriological or clinical research. Influenza is the most common virus disease of man for which adequate methods of laboratory study are available. It is a most interesting disease both clinically and epidemiologically, and the methods employed in its study are so simple as to be available to every bacteriological laboratory. A great deal may be learned from patient and painstaking study of clinical cases by the technique available, and this includes such important problems as the whereabouts of the virus during interepidemic periods, the existence and nature of a carrier state, and the relationship of influenzal infection to lobar pneumonia and other complications. These are essentially research problems which will require a great deal of careful work for their solution. Where research in influenza is being carried on, it is an easy matter to fit into the program the requirements for routine diagnosis during epidemic periods. Very little useful information will come out of a service which is geared solely to the fulfillment of requests for routine diagnosis.

REFERENCES

1. Taylor, R. M., and R. J. Chialvo, Simplified technic for inoculating into amniotic sac of chick embryos, *Proc. Soc. Exp. Biol. & Med.*, 1942. 51:328.
2. Beveridge, W. I. B., and F. M. Burnet, *The Cultivation of Viruses and Rickettsiae in the Chick Embryo*, Medical Research Council, Special Report Series No. 256 (London, H.M.S. Stationery Office, 1946).

3. Salk, J. E., A simplified procedure for titrating hemagglutinating capacity of influenza-virus and the corresponding antibody, *J. Immunol.*, 1944, 49:87.
4. Magill, T. P., and J. Y. Sugg, Physical-chemical factors in agglutination of sheep erythrocytes by influenza virus, *Proc. Soc. Exp. Biol. & Med.*, 1947, 66:89.
5. Hirst, G. K., and E. G. Pickels, A method for the titration of influenza hemagglutinins and influenza antibodies with the aid of a photoelectric densitometer, *J. Immunol.*, 1942, 45:273.
6. Nigg, C., J. H. Crowley, and D. E. Wilson, The use of chick embryo tissues and fluid as antigens in the complement fixation reaction in influenza, *J. Immunol.*, 1941, 42:51.
7. Whitman, L., A modified agglutination-inhibition test for the diagnosis of influenza, *Bull. U. S. Army Med. Dept.*, 1946, 6:777.
8. Rickard, E. R., M. Thigpen, and J. H. Crowley, The isolation of influenza A virus by the intraallantoic inoculation of chick embryos with untreated throat-washings, *J. Immunol.*, 1944, 49:263.
9. Hirst, G. K., Direct isolation of influenza virus in chick embryos, *J. Immunol.*, 1942, 45:293.

Chapter 3

THE DIAGNOSIS OF MUMPS

BY GERTRUDE HENLE AND WERNER HENLE, *The Children's Hospital of Philadelphia, Department of Pediatrics, School of Medicine, University of Pennsylvania*

DURING THE PAST FEW YEARS, it has become possible to handle mumps virus conveniently in the laboratory, chiefly because of the studies of Enders and Habel. The adaptation of the virus to the chick embryo (1), the observation of the hemagglutination phenomenon (2), and the development of complement-fixation and skin tests (3) have greatly facilitated the study of the disease in its various aspects. The brief period which has elapsed since these discoveries has not permitted, as yet, the collection of data from many outbreaks of mumps, and only a few publications on diagnostic procedures are available thus far. As a consequence, this report is limited mainly to experience gained in the Virus Laboratories of The Children's Hospital of Philadelphia.[1] The data to be presented were gathered during mumps epidemics from the fall of 1946 to the spring of 1947, in Philadelphia, Kentucky, Sweden, and Canada. It is advisable, therefore, to regard the conclusions to be drawn with the reservation that studies of epidemics in future years may not necessarily duplicate in every respect the results to be reported.

The clinical diagnosis of typical mumps, that is, of mumps parotitis, usually does not offer any difficulties, and, consequently, the assistance of the laboratory will not be required. However, in some of the more unusual manifestations of the infection, such as meningoencephalitis, orchitis, and pancreatitis, in the absence of preceding or concurrent definite involvement of the salivary glands, laboratory tests are needed for the confirmation or establishment of the diagnosis. The determination of susceptibility or resistance to mumps constitutes another problem for the diagnostic laboratory.

In order to ascertain the value of diagnostic procedures, it is obvious that they will have to be analyzed first in relation to the typical

[1] The studies described in this paper were aided by the Office of Naval Research.

disease. As in most viral infections, there exist two approaches to the laboratory diagnosis: the isolation from the patient of the etiological agent and its identification; and the demonstration of a characteristic antibody response in the patient's serum.

ISOLATION OF VIRUS

According to the available evidence (4, 5, 6), mumps virus may best be isolated in 8-day-old chick embryos by amniotic inoculation of saliva from cases of parotitis, or of spinal fluid from cases of meningo-encephalitis. The specimens should be used shortly after they have been obtained, or they should be rapidly frozen and stored in that state until injections can be made. Sufficient amounts of penicillin and streptomycin are added to the specimens of saliva so that they contain 100 to 1,000 units of each per inoculum, and the mixtures are incubated at 37°C. for thirty minutes to one hour. A hole of about 1 cm. in diameter is cut into the shell of the egg above the air sac on the side where the embryo is located. A piece of the shell membrane is removed with a forceps without rupturing the underlying allantoic sac. Through this window the embryo becomes visible within the amniotic sac and the injection is made under direct observation. The hole in the shell is sealed with scotch tape. Ten eggs are used for the first passage, since the mortality of the embryos injected with saliva may be high. After incubation of the eggs for four to seven days at 35-37°C., the amniotic fluids are tested for their capacity to agglutinate chicken red cells. Further passages are made by the same route with amniotic fluid alone, or with amniotic membranes emulsified in amniotic fluid. The isolated virus may be identified through the use of one of several techniques:

a) Complement-fixation tests with known acute and convalescent sera, using as antigen, amniotic fluid infected with the new strain;
b) Inhibition by known high-titered immune sera of hemagglutination caused by the new virus;
c) Neutralization by known immune sera of the infectivity of the new agent for chick embryos.

By means of these techniques, a number of strains of mumps virus have been isolated in this laboratory. In addition, information has been obtained as to the period of excretion of virus in the saliva of

TABLE 1

ISOLATION OF MUMPS VIRUS FROM VARIOUS CASES OF EPIDEMIC AND EXPERIMENTAL INFECTION

Patient	Disease	Material	Days after Onset	Isolation of Virus; Hemagglutination in Passages		
				1	2	3
B. F.	Parotitis	Saliva*	1, 2, & 3	—	—	—
P. I. D. 1–7	Parotitis	Saliva*	1	—	—	..
D. D.	Parotitis	Saliva	1	+	..	..
R. F.	Parotitis	Saliva	1	+	..	..
T. B.	Parotitis	Saliva	1	+	..	..
C. H.	Parotitis	Saliva	1	—	—	..
A. P.	Meningo-encephalitis	Spinal fluid	1	+	..	..
T. P.	Meningo-encephalitis	Spinal fluid	1	—	+	..
P. O.	Experimental parotitis	Saliva	1	—	+	..
F. G.	Experimental parotitis	Saliva	1	—	+	..
C. W.	Experimental parotitis	Saliva	−5	—	—	..
		Saliva	−3	—	+	..
		Saliva	0	+	..	..
		Saliva	3	+	..	..
		Saliva	7	—	—	..
M. H.	Parotitis following contact with experimental cases	Saliva	1	+	..	..
		Saliva	4	—	—	..

* These specimens were frozen twice before the test; all others were used fresh or after rapid freezing and storage at −40° C.

cases of experimental infection (7). Table 1 summarizes some of these data. As can be seen, virus was isolated from saliva of cases of experimental mumps as early as three days before, and as late as three days after, onset of disease. Leymaster and Ward (5) obtained virus from saliva as late as six days after onset of parotitis. The two spinal fluids yielding virus were withdrawn from cases of meningo-encephalitis without parotitis on the first day of illness (6). In successful isolations, hemagglutination was obtained frequently in the first passage and in the remaining ones on the second transfer. A specimen is considered negative only if three passages fail to yield hemagglutinins. These data show, then, that the diagnosis of infection with the virus of mumps by isolation of the agent can be made at the earliest in four to seven days, but requires, frequently, a longer period.

There remain many questions in regard to isolation procedures. The available data are too scanty to permit a statement as to the frequency of isolations to be expected. The results may be affected by the way a specimen is treated from the time it is obtained from the patient until it can be injected into the egg. Obviously, success or failure may depend on the properties of the epidemic strain of virus. Although the available data fail to indicate the existence of different antigenic types of mumps virus, future studies possibly may yield such evidence. By analogy with the experience gained in influenza, the results may conceivably be influenced by factors such as differences in the capacity of various strains of mumps virus to agglutinate red cells of individual chickens or of different species. These are various possibilities which hardly have been explored as yet.

THE SEROLOGICAL DIAGNOSIS OF MUMPS

For the serological diagnosis of mumps, three different techniques have been described in the literature, which could conceivably be of use: (a) the inhibition of hemagglutination (2); (b) the agglutination by specific mumps antibodies of red cells coated with mumps antigen—the Burnet test (8); and (c) the complement-fixation test (3). Of these three, we feel that only the complement-fixation test is sufficiently reliable as yet for routine diagnostic tests. Furthermore, both the inhibition of hemagglutination and the Burnet test always require the comparison of sera taken during the acute stage with specimens obtained during convalescence. The complement-fixation test, on the other hand, may yield diagnostically significant results frequently with a single serum taken in the first days of illness.

The inhibition of hemagglutination suffers from the fact that normal sera, that is, sera from susceptible individuals, will inhibit the phenomenon to some extent. Convalescent sera, on the other hand, frequently do not attain very high neutralizing titers. Thus, the difference between the acute and the convalescent sera in their capacity to inhibit hemagglutination may often be small, placing the results in the category of "doubtful" responses. As to the Burnet test, it has been found difficult in our hands to obtain stable suspensions of red cells after they have been treated with mumps virus, that is, the treated suspensions are usually autoagglutinable and, therefore, cannot be used in the test.

The complement fixation reaction has been found very useful in extensive studies by Enders and his co-workers (3, 9, 10). In the early tests antigens were derived from the infected parotid glands of monkeys. More recently they were prepared from the infected chick embryo (1, 2). An analysis in this laboratory of the complement-fixation antigens present in the chick embryo infected with a strain of mumps virus, received from Dr. Enders, revealed that there exist at least two serologically distinct antigens; one is linked with the virus particle, and may be called "Virus" or "V antigen"; the other is smaller in size and may be termed "Soluble" or "S antigen" (11). Various data concerning the properties of these two antigens are recorded in Table 2. The antigens presently used in our laboratory consist of infected

TABLE 2

PROPERTIES OF V AND S ANTIGENS

Antigen	Source	Treatment	Infectivity for Chick Embryos ID 50/ml.	Hemagglutination Titer	Complement Fixation with Convalescent Serum Absorbed with		
					Native	V	S
V	Allantoic fluid	..	$10^{7.8}$	1:1536	++++	0	++++
		Supernate 20,000 r.p.m.	$10^{5.6}$	1:8	0	..	..
S	Allantoic membrane	..	$10^{5.8}$	0	++++	..	..
		Supernate 20,000 r.p.m.	$10^{2.9}$	0	++++	++++	0

dialyzed allantoic fluid (V antigen), and a 20 percent suspension of allantoic membrane, clarified by high-speed centrifugation at 20,000 r.p.m. for 20 minutes (S antigen). The infectivity in both preparations is inactivated by ultraviolet irradiation, and merthiolate is added as preservative. The antigens are stable for several months at 4°C. They are standardized for the complement-fixation test by optimal titration technique, and that amount of antigen is used which gives the highest antibody titer with known convalescent sera.

A control antigen is prepared from normal allantoic sacs according to the technique used for the infected membranes. Some human sera may fix complement to a varying extent with this material. This property of the sera is independent of the Wassermann reaction (12). It may frequently be decreased by inactivating the sera for a second time at 60°C. for twenty minutes (3). Absorption of the serum with cytoplasmic particles of normal allantoic membranes or with sheep erythrocytes removes the nonspecific reactions without reducing the specific antibodies in the serum (12). The latter procedure is employed routinely now in this laboratory.

An analysis of sera from experimental and epidemic cases of mumps has shown that antibodies against the soluble antigen usually appear before anti-V, and that anti-S may have reached high levels at the time signs of illness have developed (12). Illustrations for this observation are shown in Table 3. These relationships have been encountered in the majority of cases studied, but, on occasion, exceptions occur in that anti-V may appear simultaneously with or even prior to anti-S. During convalescence antibodies against both V and S antigens show high titers, anti-V usually exceeding anti-S. Subsequently, the titers decrease, anti-S at a faster rate, as a rule, than anti-V. Thus, several years after infection, antibodies against the V antigen only may be left, whereas antibodies against S may no longer be demonstrable (Table 3). In some cases both antibodies may have disappeared from the serum (13).

These data indicate that both the V and S antigens have their place in diagnostic procedures. If only the S antigen is used, one may find, not infrequently, that the serum taken in the acute stage of mumps already shows high antibody levels, and no significant increase in titer will become apparent in subsequent serum specimens. Under these circumstances, a definite laboratory diagnosis cannot be made, since the finding of a high antibody level per se ($>1:96$ according to Enders' technique [3], or $>1:16$ by our calculations [12]) implies a recent but not necessarily current infection with mumps virus. With the use of the V antigen alone, this situation does not obtain because of the somewhat delayed development of antibodies against this antigen, so that an increase in titer can be measured in practically all cases. However, five days or more are required in most patients before a definite rise becomes apparent. If one employs both V and S anti-

TABLE 3

COMPLEMENT-FIXING ANTIBODIES TO THE SOLUBLE AND VIRUS ANTIGENS AT VARYING TIMES AFTER THE ONSET OF MUMPS

Case Number	Onset of Disease	Days after Onset	Antibody Titers — Initial Dilutions		Supernate of Normal Membranes
			vs. SOLUBLE ANTIGEN	vs. VIRUS ANTIGEN	
H 49	3/12/47 Parotitis	1	1:2	0	0
		3	1:24	<1:2	0
		5	1:32	1:3	0
		9	1:64	1:24	0
47	2/28/47 Parotitis	5	1:16	<1:2	0
		6	1:32	1:3	Tr.
		11	1:32	1:32	0
		15	1:64	1:64	0
M.D.	5/17/47 Meningo-encephalitis	2	1:64	1:4	0
		14	1:64	1:64	0
M 27	1944 Parotitis	2½ yr.	1:2	1:8	0
H 8	1942 Parotitis	5 yr.	<1:4	1:32	0

gens, a presumptive diagnosis of infection with mumps virus may be made in many instances in the first few days of the disease. The finding of a high titer of anti-S, and of low levels or lack of anti-V, is considered diagnostically significant for the first days of illness. This situation has permitted the recognition of mumps meningo-encephalitis in the absence of parotitis, as early as two days after onset, as in case M.D. in Table 3 (12). In some instances, the early serum does not reveal such a characteristic picture. In that case, the diagnosis depends on the demonstration of rises in antibodies against V and S. If the meningo-encephalitis occurs as a late complication after an earlier, inapparent infection, or after indefinite manifestations of infection, both antibodies may be at high levels in the first available serum, and no further rises will become apparent. In these cases only a suggestive laboratory diagnosis can be made.

In order to determine whether or not an individual is resistant to mumps, two tests may be used, the complement-fixation reaction (3, 10, 13) and the skin test (3, 14). As far as the complement-fixation test is concerned, the sera of human beings who have experienced either apparent or inapparent infections with mumps virus at some time in the past will frequently react with the V antigen, but often no longer with S. A few may fail to show any reactions. Thus, a positive complement-fixation test gives reasonable assurance of immunity, whereas a negative reaction does not necessarily imply susceptibility. This interpretation is borne out by the observation that in an outbreak of mumps in a school all cases occurred among those children whose sera failed to react with the V antigen at the beginning of the epidemic (13). On the other hand, a few children in this serological class escaped apparent or inapparent infection during the period of the epidemic. It is impossible to decide at present whether this result is an indication of a less intimate exposure of some of the children to the infectious agent, or whether these subjects possessed levels of anti-V too low to measure but still sufficient to protect against reinfection, or, finally, whether an antibody other than anti-V, which is not discovered by the currently used complement-fixation technique, is responsible for resistance to mumps. These problems require further elucidation.

For the determination of dermal hypersensitivity Enders and coworkers (3, 14) used in the early studies skin-test antigens prepared from the parotid glands of infected monkeys. More recently, inactivated infected allantoic fluids have been employed (15). Following intradermal injection of these antigens most *immune* individuals will respond within twenty-four to forty-eight hours with erythema and induration measuring, as a rule, in excess of 15 mm. in diameter. The *susceptible* subjects fail to respond, or show reactions of less than 15 mm. in diameter. Individuals who deny a past experience of mumps show dermal hypersensitivity in about 50 percent in the case of adults, and in about 25 percent in children; these figures indicate the relative frequency of inapparent infections. Exceptions to the suggested interpretation of skin reactions are encountered not infrequently. Children with definite histories of mumps are found to react less intensively than adults. Not all patients develop dermal hypersensitivity; some may lose it in the course of several years, and, on the other hand, cases of mumps occur among subjects who previously yielded positive skin reactions. These various observations tend to decrease somewhat the reliability of the skin test.

In comparing the results of the skin test with those of the complement-fixation reaction, discrepancies become apparent in a number of instances. Not every individual reacting with the V antigen will give a positive skin test, and, conversely, not every subject showing dermal hypersensitivity will yield a positive complement-fixation reaction. These data indicate clearly that the two tests complement each other, and it is suggested that both techniques be used at present where highest possible accuracy is desired in the determination of susceptibility to mumps.

REFERENCES

1. Habel, K., Cultivation of mumps virus in the developing chick embryo and its application to studies of immunity to mumps in man, *Pub. Health Rep.*, 1945, 60:201.
2. Levens, J. H., and J. F. Enders, The hemagglutinative properties of amniotic fluid from embryonated eggs infected with mumps virus, *Science*, 1945, 102:117.
3. Enders, J. F., S. Cohen, and L. W. Kane, Immunity in mumps, II: The development of complement-fixing antibody and dermal hypersensitivity in human beings following mumps, *J. Exp. Med.*, 1945, 81:119.
4. Beveridge, W. I. B., P. E. Lind, and S. G. Anderson, Mumps, I: Isolation and cultivation of the virus in the chick embryo, *Australian J. Exp. Biol. & Med. Sci.*, 1946, 24:15.
5. Leymaster, G. R., and T. G. Ward, Direct isolation of mumps virus in chick embryos, *Proc. Soc. Exp. Biol. & Med.*, 1947, 65:346.
6. Henle, G., and C. L. McDougall, Mumps meningo-encephalitis; isolation in chick embryos of virus from spinal fluid of a patient, *Proc. Soc. Exp. Biol. & Med.*, 1947, 66:209.
7. Henle, G., W. Henle, K. K. Wendell, and P. Rosenberg, Isolation of mumps virus from human beings with induced apparent or inapparent infections, *J. Exp. Med.*, 1948, 88:223.
8. Burnet, F. M., Modification of human red cells by virus action, III: A sensitive test for mumps antibody in human serum by the agglutination of human red cells coated with virus antigen, *Brit. J. Exp. Path.*, 1946, 27:244.
9. Kane, L. W., and J. F. Enders, Immunity in mumps, III: The complement fixation test as an aid in the diagnosis of mumps meningo-encephalitis, *J. Exp. Med.*, 1945, 81:137.
10. Maris, E. P., J. F. Enders, J. Stokes, Jr., and L. W. Kane, Immunity in mumps; the correlation of the presence of complement-fixing antibody and resistance to mumps in human beings, *J. Exp. Med.*, 1946, 84:323.
11. Henle, G., W. Henle, and S. Harris, The serological differentiation of mumps complement-fixation antigens, *Proc. Soc. Exp. Biol. & Med.*, 1947, 64:290.

12. Henle, G., S. Harris, and W. Henle, The reactivity of various human sera with mumps complement fixation antigens, *J. Exp. Med.*, 1948, 88:133.
13. Henle, G., W. Henle, and S. Harris, The use of complement-fixation technic in the analysis of two institutional outbreaks of mumps, *Pediatrics*, 1948, 1:593.
14. Enders, J. F., L. W. Kane, E. P. Maris, and J. Stokes, Jr., Immunity in mumps, V: The correlation of the presence of dermal hypersensitivity and resistance to mumps, *J. Exp. Med.*, 1946, 84:341.
15. Davis, H. E., J. Stokes, Jr., J. F. Enders, G. Henle, and E. P. Maris, Studies on active immunization against mumps. (Not yet published.)

Chapter 4

THE DIAGNOSIS OF INFECTIONS CAUSED BY THE PSITTACOSIS–LYMPHOGRANULOMA GROUP OF VIRUSES (INCLUDING TRACHOMA AND INCLUSION BLENNORRHEA)

By Geoffrey Rake, *The Squibb Institute for Medical Research*

The group of agents producing diseases whose diagnosis is considered here, the Chlamydozoaceae (1), is one of particular interest from the taxonomic and evolutionary point of view. It will, however, be sufficient, as an introduction to this discussion, to draw attention to the fact that these agents are sufficiently large to be seen by the light microscope, where they reveal themselves to be coccoid in shape; that with the electron microscope their morphology is quite characteristic and unlike that of any other microorganism of which I am cognizant (2); that they stain with most of the ordinary aniline dyes; that they are apparently obligate intracytoplasmic parasites and have never been grown in artificial media; and finally, that all members are susceptible, to one degree or another, to at least one chemotherapeutic substance, whether of natural or of synthetic origin. These agents have been found as pathogens in mammals, including man, various rodents, and cats, and in birds of many genera; and while the present discussion will cover chiefly those which are capable of producing disease in man, namely, the agents of psittacosis and ornithosis, lymphogranuloma venereum, trachoma, and inclusion blennorrhea, reference will be made on more than one occasion to information which has been obtained by working with other members of the group.

PSITTACOSIS[1] AND ORNITHOSIS

General statement. With the success of the sulfonamide drugs there emerged a relatively new clinical entity which is now generally known as primary atypical pneumonia. This nonbacterial pneumonitis undoubtedly includes many diseases of diverse etiology, amongst which

[1] The author wishes to acknowledge his indebtedness to Dr. K. F. Meyer for much of the material which is discussed under the subject of psittacosis. (See chapter on psittacosis in textbook, *Diagnostic Procedures for Virus and Rickettsial Diseases* [3].)

one may mention the agents of Q fever and influenza, besides, of course, the still ill-defined agent of atypical pneumonia itself. In recent years it has been clear that psittacosis and psittacosoid agents play some role as etiological factors. That this may be increasingly true in the future is suggested by the apparently increasing incidence of the psittacosis viruses in flocks of domesticated or semidomesticated birds, such as chickens, ducks, and pigeons, as well as in many wild birds such as fulmar petrels, gulls and waders, which have been demonstrated to be extensively infected by many investigators, including Meyer and his co-workers (4, 5), and Smadel and his co-workers (6) in this country, Coles in South Africa (7), and Andrewes and Mills in England (8). Thus the sense of security which was formerly enjoyed by those who did not associate themselves with any of the pet birds, whether parrots, finches, or doves, is now known to be false.

Clinical manifestations. The onset of psittacosis is often acute and is associated with general malaise, headache, fever, chills, and vomiting. The fever tends to be remittent but persisting. Compared to the high temperature, the pulse is relatively slow. There is nonproductive cough, but physical signs develop slowly, are often slight, and may be of a transient nature. X-ray examinations frequently show patchy involvement of the lungs. Sputum, however, tends to be scanty, an important point from the diagnostic point of view, since an expectorant may have to be given in order to obtain sufficient sputum for diagnostic purposes. The disease, particularly with some of the strains of psittacosis agent which have been described and in individuals over the age of 40, has a high mortality, but there are no characteristics to set it clearly apart from other forms of pneumonia. Psittacosis must be considered in any case of pneumonitis not responding to sulfonamide therapy, particularly in those in which a history of contact with birds, whether the latter were sick or not, can be obtained.

Diagnosis. Because of certain complications connected with the methods for serological diagnosis usually employed in this disease, the certain diagnosis of this infection cannot be made without (*a*) the isolation and identification of the agent and (*b*) the demonstration of an increase in serum antibodies between the acute phase of the illness and the period of recovery.

Isolation. In order that one may discuss intelligently the isolation of the virus it is necessary to describe briefly the pathology of psittacosis. As has already been indicated, this disease is primarily a pneumonitis with scattered lobular areas of consolidation and often with pleurisy, but usually without much exudate in the bronchioles. In man the spleen may be enlarged and soft, and central focal necroses are found in the liver. Septicemias with plentiful virus in the blood occur more commonly than was formerly recognized. In birds the pulmonary changes are often more extreme and a seropurulent exudate is not uncommon. Both spleen and liver tend to be greatly enlarged, and the areas of necrosis in the liver can often be seen with the naked eye. One should note that all of the infections under consideration in this section are characterized by a high frequency of latent cases in which the virus may be carried without overt signs of the disease. In such cases, particularly in birds with psittacosis, the only lesion to be observed is an enlarged spleen and even that may be lacking. It may require an intercurrent infection, a dietary deficiency or extreme physical conditions to bring on signs of overt disease. The commonest material presented for isolation from human cases is sputum, blood or pleural fluid, or fragments of lung, spleen, or liver taken at autopsy. In the case of birds, whole cadavers may be submitted, and virus should be looked for particularly in the spleen and lungs.

Precautions must be taken in the handling of material which may possibly contain the psittacosis virus. Many members of this group of agents are extremely infectious for man and produce a disease which in the past has had a high mortality rate. It is certainly inadvisable for material which may contain the active virus to be worked with in a routine laboratory; and even those individuals who are accustomed to handling members of this group, when working with unknown material which may contain new strains of the agent, should take great care to prevent dissemination of infected material in dust or in droplet form, to protect themselves from any chance infection, particularly by the upper respiratory tract, and to dispose of any material used efficiently and completely.

Many of the materials discussed above, which may be presented for the isolation of the virus, can be expected to be free from bacterial contamination, but others, as, for example, sputum, will probably be contaminated with bacteria and must be treated accordingly. For this purpose, probably the best technique includes the use of chemotherapeutic substances which either have no effect on these agents *in vitro* or work only in high concentrations. Amongst material suggested for these purposes are combinations of tyrothricin, sulfadiazine, and streptomycin on the one hand (3), or of penicillin and streptomycin on the other (9). Satisfactory results have been obtained with both of these mixtures.

Submitted material should first be examined to determine whether bodies characteristic of this group of viruses, or other pathogenic agents, can be seen on direct microscopic examination of smears. Smears are prepared from sputum or body fluids, or from emulsions of tissues, and may be stained by any one of several methods, of which perhaps the best are those of Macchiavello, or the so-called rapid Giemsa (9). Under suitable circumstances the characteristic spherical elementary bodies of psittacosis may be seen. These measure approximately 350 mμ in diameter and are, therefore, readily visible with a good light microscope. They appear singly or in groups, either extracellularly or within the cytoplasm of tissue cells, particularly monocytes. In particularly favorable circumstances, especially in heavily infected tissues of birds, larger forms of the bodies, the so-called initial bodies, which measure up to 1,000 mμ in diameter, can be seen, or inclusion bodies may be made out within the infected cells of the host.

However, all of these morphological characteristics are common to every member of the Chlamydozoaceae, and for this reason, isolation must be achieved. The selection of animals for isolation of the virus requires consideration. Perhaps the best animal is still the laboratory mouse, but extreme precautions must be taken to avoid false positive findings. Thus, an increasing number of herds of these animals have been found to be infected with one member of this group, namely, the agent of murine pneumonitis (10). Furthermore, as studies from Australia have apparently shown, occasional spontaneous infection of a herd of mice may occur with an agent indistinguishable from that of psittacosis (11). In any laboratory, therefore, which expects to be called upon to carry out isolation experiments in this group of agents, a source of mice should be kept on hand and tested at suitable intervals for the possible occurrence of spontaneous infection. This may be done by blind passage of lung material or by the provocation of the disease by the intranasal installation of sterile broth into anesthetized animals and again the passage of any pneumonic areas obtained into clean mice. No mammal is more valuable than the mouse because all others are less susceptible and of greater initial and continuing expense. Furthermore, it is now recognized that agents of the psittacosis-lymphogranuloma group may occur spontaneously in rodents other than mice.

The high rate of overt or latent infection of birds, particularly in psittacine birds, pigeons, and finches, does not in general recommend them for isolation procedures. However, pigeons have a usefulness in distinguishing strains of ornithosis from those of psittacosis. Strains of the former are far more virulent by the intracerebral route in these birds than are strains of the latter (32). Meyer (3) points out that ricebirds or Java finches would be excellent but for their prohibitively high price. It is also to be noted that infected birds are more dangerous to those carrying out the experimental studies than are infected rodents. The chicken embryo offers many advantages. To the present time I know of no case in which any of this group of agents have been found spontaneously infecting the embryonated chicken embryo; the egg is easy to handle; and it is cheap. Possible disadvantages are, first, the extremely high susceptibility of the embryonated egg, particularly when the yolk-sac route of inoculation is used, to even a minute number of bacteria in the inoculum, and, second, the observation that the egg may be less susceptible than is the mouse when the isolation of the new strains direct from birds or mammals is concerned (12). This, of course, does not hold, particularly if the yolk-sac route of inoculation is used, once the agent has been established in the laboratory. At that time yolk-sac inoculation will detect virus in concentrations at least one-tenth that which can be detected by any infection in mice.

As far as the route of inoculation is concerned, intraperitoneal injection is suggested in the mouse. The symptoms produced depend upon the strain of the virus and the amount contained in the inoculum. In general, the mice show ruffled fur, conjunctival exudate, and distended abdomen; these symptoms appear anywhere from two to fifteen days after inoculation. In cases where only small amounts of virus have been present, the symptoms are transient and may be missed. In those cases where no strain of the agent is established with certainty in the first passage, and no other pathogen has been incriminated, at least two blind passages should be carried out, killing surviving mice at twenty to thirty days and passing spleen and liver to fresh mice. Gross lesions and elementary bodies should be sought for in lung, liver, and spleen. Elementary bodies may also be present in peritoneal or pleural exudates. Isolation by intranasal or intracerebral inoculation of mice should be carried out as a supplementary procedure to isolate strains of ornithosis which may not infect by the intraperitoneal route or infect only if inoculated in large doses.

In the embryonated egg the yolk-sac method of inoculation is probably the best, but some workers have utilized inoculation either onto the chorioallantoic membrane or into the allantoic sac. If the yolk-sac route of inoculation is used, six-day embryos should be employed and, from the second day after inoculation onward, the egg should be candled twice a day. Death usually occurs in from three to eight days and is preceded by a period of sluggishness, at which time the embryo should be sacrificed and the yolk sac harvested. Smears of specifically infected yolk cells will show a plentiful supply of elementary bodies. In the case of embryonated eggs, as with mice, it may be necessary to carry out two or three blind passages, with a tenfold suspension of yolk sac in broth, in order to establish the agent.

If it is desired to carry out further microscopic studies either on the original material or on tissues from experimental animals, fixed paraffin sections may be prepared and stained to advantage with either Giemsa's stain or Noble's stain (13), but these probably have little place in techniques undertaken purely for the identification of one of this group of agents.

Identification. Even if the primary isolation has not been made in the embryonated chick egg, it should be transferred to this animal by the yolk-sac route of inoculation as soon as possible, to obtain adequate amounts of virus. Identification of the agent is possible by means of at least two serological tests. The first of these is the toxin-antitoxin neutralization test (14). The agents of psittacosis and ornithosis, in common with other agents of this group that have been studied, produce a specific toxic factor, and the lethal effect of this can be neutralized by homologous antitoxin but not by normal or heterologous sera. Such antitoxin is produced in rabbits or chickens. The neutralization can be carried out *in vivo* by passive transfer of protection, or *in vitro*. For practical purposes the latter technique is preferable. The second specific method lies in the use of chicken neutralizing antisera as described by Hilleman (15). Unlike antisera prepared in mammals, particularly in rabbits, which fail to give satisfactory and clear-cut neutralization against any of the agents of this group, sera prepared by intraperitoneal inoculation of chickens give satisfactory neutralization with good but not complete specificity. Such chicken sera also give agglutination of the homologous antigens, as do rabbit sera, but the specificity of such agglutination methods has not been demonstrated. In general, the complement-fixation test, even with known sera, cannot be used because of the marked cross reaction that occurs between homologous and heterologous antigens and antisera with this test in this group of agents (16). However, the picture here is still in process of clarification, since, for example, Eddie and Francis (17) have described sera of pigeons infected with psittacosis which gave no complement fixation with antigen prepared from lymphogranuloma venereum, and recently Wall (18) has described complement-fixing antigens obtained from mice infected with lymphogranuloma venereum which reacted with the homologous antigen but not with one prepared from virus of psittacosis.

Quite apart from the above specific serological tests, there are methods by which the agent can be distinguished from other described members of the group. These depend on sulfonamide susceptibility and tissue tropisms. The agents of lymphogranuloma venereum, mouse pneumonitis, trachoma, inclusion blennorrhea, and some strains of psittacosis are susceptible to sulfonamide therapy. The agents of trachoma and inclusion blennorrhea have not been transmitted to any laboratory animals. The agent of psittacosis infects mice intraperitoneally, but that of lymphogranuloma venereum does not. The agent of mouse pneumonitis fails to infect mice intracerebrally, but that of lymphogranuloma venereum does infect by this route.

Serological diagnosis of the disease. As was originally demonstrated by Bedson (19), serum from mammals or birds infected with the agent of psittacosis fixed complement in the presence of the homologous antigen and agglutinated the elementary bodies. The former test may be used for presumptive diagnosis of the infection when the agent has not been isolated and also for field surveys of flocks of birds or herds of animals thought to be infected with one or another member of the group. Several methods of carrying out the complement-fixation test have been employed and are adequately described in the literature (3, 9). Satisfactory antigen may be prepared from spleens or lungs of infected mice, from tissue culture on agar slants (20), or from infected yolk sac. The same antigens, particularly the last, may be used for the preparation of suspensions of elementary bodies for agglutination tests.

The complement-fixation test is highly sensitive, but unless the results obtained are interpreted with caution they may give rise to considerable error. Such error occurs from three causes, particularly if the egg-yolk antigen is used; two of these sources of error can be eliminated by the use of normal antigen control prepared from the same tissue as that used in preparing the specific antigen. Such control antigen will eliminate from consideration those individuals who are sensitive to normal yolk sac and whose sera, therefore, react nonspecifically with both specific and normal antigen. It will also eliminate that group of syphilitic individuals who, particularly in the early stages of their disease, show a similar nonspecific fixation with yolk-sac antigens. Such nonspecific fixation usually disappears in the later stages of the syphilitic infection or after cure. The third source of error, and the one most likely to cause difficulties, depends on the fact, already mentioned, that there is considerable cross reaction in the complement-fixation test between antigens or antibodies prepared with the various members of this group of agents. Furthermore, because of the high degree of frequency with which a persistent carrier state is set up, even in the absence of acute infection at any time, complement-fixing antibodies may be present in high titer without being significant in the case of which the diagnosis is in question. Under these circumstances, when both acute and convalescent sera are available, a significant rise in complement-fixing antibodies will implicate one of this group of agents as the etiological factor, but in the majority of cases it will not be possible to state from this evidence alone which of the agents is involved. The reason for the occasional occurrence of specific complement-fixation tests which has been mentioned above, in contradistinction to the usual broad group reaction, has not been sufficiently investigated. When only convalescent serum is available, positive fixation even of high degree can be interpreted only as showing that the individual has been exposed at some time in the past to one of the members of this group.

As will be pointed out later, the intradermal test with antigen prepared from lymphogranuloma venereum is considerably more specific than is the complement-fixation test. Though the reason for this is still under investigation, it seems possible that it is the involvement of different antigen-antibody systems (21). The intradermal test has not been used in psittacosis to the same degree that it has in lymphogranuloma venereum, principally because in psittacosis one is dealing with an acute infection and in lymphogranuloma, with a chronic and sustained disease. Nevertheless, it seems probable that more careful attention to the intradermal test in infections with this group of agents would prove valuable.

Also remaining to be fully elucidated is the help in diagnosis which may be obtained from the utilization of acute and convalescent sera in the toxin-antitoxin reaction. In this case also preliminary results have suggested a field of usefulness (14).

LYMPHOGRANULOMA VENEREUM

Clinical manifestations. As the name implies, this next disease is one of venereal origin, and the lesions from which the agent must be isolated are usually, but not invariably, in the genital or anal region. The disease in its most characteristic form begins with a primary lesion—a small transient vesicle on the genitalia which is frequently unnoticed. This is followed within one to seven weeks by pain and swelling of the regional lymph nodes, which, if untreated, suppurate and drain through the overlying skin. The whole episode may run its course without fever, but this is not always the case. In rare instances there may be acute septicemic episodes at the onset, and later meningitis or pneumonitis. The primary lesion may also be in the mouth and is often destructive in this site, or in the eye, where again it produces a highly destructive lesion clinically distinguishable with difficulty from acute trachoma. In both sexes spread of the disease to deeper lymph nodes or primary ano-rectal implantation leads to chronic elephantiasis of the genitalia, and to fistulae and rectal stricture.

Isolation. In many cases bacterial contamination of the material available for diagnosis exists. Thus, the commonest material presented for isolation procedures is pus from an inguinal bubo, or biopsy material from buboes or rectal and anal lesions. In the case of bubo pus, the rate of contamination with bacteria is approximately 20 percent (12, 22); in the case of biopsy material from the ano-genital region it is usually, if not invariably, much higher. Blood, spinal fluid, or lymph-node material, where no tracking to the outside has occurred, may be expected to be sterile. In any case in which there is any possibility of bacterial contamination, the material should be treated with antibiotic mixtures such as those discussed under psittacosis.

As was pointed out for psittacosis, individuals working with material possibly lymphogranulomatous must bear in mind its pathogenic nature. Many cases of laboratory infection occurred before strict precautions were adopted, and the disease, if not lethal, can be highly unpleasant. Vaccination has not proved efficacious. Strict precautions must be observed.

Submitted material may be examined for bodies characteristic of lymphogranuloma venereum (which resemble those of psittacosis), but the probability of finding these in direct smear is even less in lymphogranuloma than it is in psittacosis. Morever, since, as has been pointed out, the morphological characteristics are common to every member of this group, one must proceed with isolation. This can be carried out in mice by the intracerebral route or in chicken embryos, preferably by the yolk-sac route. The same arguments for or against mice or chicken embryos hold for lymphogranuloma as were given for psittacosis, although if the intracerebral route of inoculation and passage in the mice is used exclusively, the chance of picking up a spontaneous virus of this group is very low. In the presence of large amounts of virus, specifically infected mice will show, beginning on the second, third, or a later day, ruffled fur, loss of weight, and a hunchback gait; but, particularly in the first passage, no symptoms may develop and blind passage should be resorted to. The number of blind passages to be made is open to question, but in our experience, if a strain of lymphogranuloma venereum is not established by the second passage, no strains will ultimately be derived. In the case of the yolk-sac route of inoculation, careful smearing of yolk sacs harvested six days after inoculation may reveal the characteristic bodies of the virus even in the absence of any signs of disease in the embryo. In the case of isolation by use of the yolk sac, blind passage should also be resorted to where necessary to establish the strain. Material from yolk sac or mouse brain should be smeared and stained by the same methods as those described for psittacosis.

Identification. The identification of the isolated agent may be proceeded with in the manner described for psittacosis. As in the case of that virus, the complement-fixation test has limited value, although, as has already been pointed out, Wall (18) has shown that antisera from mice recovered from lymphogranuloma will not give cross fixation with psittacosis antigen. It is possible that such sera may be of use.

In those cases in which successful isolation is not achieved, positive diagnosis may be made through the inactivation of the submitted material with heat or formalin and its utilization as a skin-test antigen in known cases of lymphogranuloma venereum (22). This is particularly easy with pus from buboes. Cases of lymphogranuloma will react in the same manner to this antigen as to the skin-test antigens usually employed, if the unknown samples contain the inactivated agent or its soluble antigen.

Immunological diagnosis of the disease. The classical method of diagnosis for lymphogranuloma venereum depends on an intradermal sensitivity reaction to an antigen containing inactivated agent or its soluble antigen. Today the diagnostic material for this test is usually prepared from heavily infected yolk sacs, and a control intradermal test is run with material prepared similarly from normal yolk sacs (23, 24). This yolk-sac antigen is more sensitive than those previously prepared from mouse brain (25) or even from human bubo pus (26). As was pointed out under psittacosis, the skin reaction in this group of diseases is considerably more specific than is the complement-fixation test and indeed appears to be due to a different antigen-antibody system (21). Rare examples of cross sensitivity with the intradermal test have been described in some cases of pneumonitis due to psittacosoid viruses (16).

Comments concerning the complement-fixation test in lymphogranuloma venereum parallel those already made for psittacosis. The test is easy to perform; the results are easy to read; and the test is more sensitive than the intradermal. The difficulties occur in the interpretation of these results. At least as far as the antigen for lymphogranuloma venereum is concerned, the use of the phenolized enhanced antigen described by Nigg and her co-workers (27) avoids many, if not all, of the nonspecific reactions which occur with sera from the early stages of syphilis, as has been discussed under psittacosis. As with psittacosis, the latent form and carrier state in lymphogranuloma venereum are of very frequent occurrence (28). Positive complement-fixation tests or even positive intradermal tests do not imply, therefore, that the disease episode under consideration is necessarily due to this agent or even to one of the group. It may merely imply past experience with such an agent. Of more significance is a difference in degree of intradermal sensitivity or a rise in serum antibodies between examinations in the acute and convalescent stages of the disease or at intervals during convalescence.

As in psittacosis, the value to be obtained from the utilization of acute and convalescent sera in the toxin-antitoxin reaction in lymphogranuloma venereum remains to be fully elucidated, but preliminary results have suggested possible usefulness for this test (14).

TRACHOMA AND INCLUSION BLENNORRHEA[2]

That the agents of trachoma and inclusion blennorrhea are related to the psittacosis-lymphogranuloma group is suggested by their morphology, by their susceptibility to certain antibiotic and synthetic drugs, and by the fact that many cases of either of these diseases demonstrate complement-fixing antibodies to antigens of the group, as, for example, that of lymphogranuloma venereum (30).

Trachoma, a disease of world-wide distribution, attacks the conjunctiva and cornea so severely as to produce poor vision or even blindness as an end result. The onset may be acute or gradual. If untreated, the disease runs a chronic course for as long as fifty years. It is stated that in young children a spontaneous cure rate may run as high as 30 percent. No matter how prolonged the course of the disease, there is rarely, if ever, any spread beyond the conjunctiva. Inclusion blennorrhea, although often thought of only as a disease of the conjunctivae, also affects the genital mucous membranes and may well be primarily a venereal disease. The genital infection, however, is usually very mild, and the disease most often comes to notice as a

[2] The author wishes to acknowledge the kind help received of Dr. Phillips Thygeson in the preparation of this section of the discussion. (See chapters on trachoma and inclusion blennorrhea in textbook, *Diagnostic Procedures for Virus and Rickettsial Diseases* [29].)

self-limited conjunctivitis (neonatal blennorrhea or swimming-pool conjunctivitis) which clears up spontaneously in all cases without any of the serious sequelae of trachoma.

Clinical features and diagnosis. The early acute phase of trachoma is characterized by a papillary hypertrophy of the conjunctiva, together with abundant conjunctival exudate containing large numbers of neutrophiles. Follicular hypertrophy is also characteristic of the chronic phase. The cornea is involved simultaneously with the conjunctiva, and the early subepithelial infiltration proceeds to corneal ulceration and cicatrization, with diminished vision or blindness. In trachoma the upper portions of the conjunctiva and cornea are more involved than the lower; in inclusion blennorrhea the reverse is true, and this feature is of diagnostic significance. In most instances trachoma can be diagnosed on clinical features alone.

Laboratory diagnosis. These agents are not so dangerous to work with as are those of psittacosis and lymphogranuloma venereum. However, it is advisable to wear glasses or goggles for all work involving potentially infectious material, and more than ordinary cleanliness of the hands should always be maintained. The elementary and initial bodies of trachoma or inclusion blennorrhea resemble those of psittacosis or lymphogranuloma venereum, described above. An important feature in the differential diagnosis of trachoma and inclusion blennorrhea from lymphogranuloma venereum in the conjunctiva lies in the fact that the inclusion bodies of trachoma and inclusion blennorrhea are embedded in a matrix which takes the stains for glycogen (31). The inclusion bodies or plaques and vesicles of lymphogranuloma venereum, psittacosis, or the other agents already discussed, do not stain for glycogen and may, therefore, be differentiated. The iodine stain of Rice (31) is particularly useful in bringing out the glycogen matrix, which appears reddish-brown and is easily recognizable even under low magnification. The number of inclusion bodies bears a relationship to the clinical severity of the disease in trachoma, and in the acute stage of the disease as many as 20 per cent of the conjunctival epithelial cells may be affected. In the chronic stage of the disease careful search may be required before inclusions can be demonstrated.

Isolation. It has not been possible to grow the agents of either trachoma or inclusion blennorrhea in tissue culture or on the embryonated chicken's egg. Moreover, no successful passage has been demonstrated in any of the ordinary laboratory animals. For experimental purposes it is possible to transmit either disease to chimpanzees, baboons, or *Macaca mulatta* monkeys, in that order of satisfactoriness as far as the resultant disease is concerned. However, such animal transmission has no value as a diagnostic procedure.

For microscopic preparations one should use either epithelial scrapings or material expressed from the hypertrophied follicles. Biopsy material is of little value. For the microscopic demonstration of the virus bodies or inclusions of trachoma, scrapings from the upper tarsus or upper fornix should be made with a platinum spatula after application of a local anesthetic. Virus bodies will be most frequent from the area of greatest disease activity. The scrapings are placed on clean slides, fixed, and stained. Staining methods to be used are those already described for psittacosis and lymphogranuloma venereum; of particular value are those of Giemsa and Macchiavello. As has already been pointed out, the Rice stain may be used for the demonstration of glycogen in the inclusion bodies. Differentiation of inclusion bodies must be made from a number of pseudo-inclusions which are apt to occur in conjunctival scrapings. These include nuclear material, or pigment in the case of heavily pigmented individuals.

Epithelial scrapings as such cannot be used to differentiate between trachoma and inclusion blennorrhea. For this purpose material expressed from the hypertrophied follicles should be used. This expressed material is stained with Giemsa stain. The material from the follicles of trachoma is characteristically soft, gelatinous, and necrotic, in contrast to the hard material obtained from follicular conjunctivitis. The material in trachoma is therefore easily expressed. In inclusion blennorrhea, the material is so difficult to set free that in some instances the whole follicle must be literally torn from the conjunctiva. In trachoma microscopic examination of the expressed material reveals numerous macrophages; numerous pale-staining, large, mononuclear cells, probably lymphoblasts; a large amount of cell debris; and a few scattered plasma cells and lymphocytes. In the material from inclusion conjunctivitis, one finds few macrophages and these tend to be smaller than those of trachoma; little, if any, cellular debris; and, as the predominant cytological feature, small lymphocytes.

As far as the cytological secretion in trachoma is concerned, the cells are predominantly neutrophilic, as has been pointed out, and this fact helps to differentiate the condition from follicular conjunctivitis due to such viruses as that of epidemic keratoconjunctivitis or herpes simplex, both of which produce a mononuclear cell reaction.

Serological procedure. No serological procedures of diagnostic importance have yet been developed for trachoma or inclusion blennorrhea. As has been pointed out, it is possible to demonstrate complement-fixing antibodies for antigens of the psittacosis-lymphogranuloma group in low titer in sera from cases of trachoma and inclusion blennorrhea. The titers tend to be higher in the more chronic cases of trachoma, and it would seem probable that the low titers usually observed can be explained on the basis of the limited extent of the disease and also, particularly in the case of inclusion blennorrhea, on its limited duration.

REFERENCES

1. Bergey, D. H., *Manual of Determinative Bacteriology.* 6th ed. Baltimore, 1948.
2. (a) Rake, G., H. Rake, D. Hamre, and V. Groupé, Electron micrographs of the agent of feline pneumonitis, *Proc. Soc. Exp. Biol. & Med.*, 1946, 63:489.
   (b) Hamre, D., H. Rake, and G. Rake, Morphological and other characteristics of the agent of feline pneumonitis grown in the allantoic cavity of the chick embryo, *J. Exp. Med.*, 1947, 86:1.
3. Meyer, K. F., *Diagnostic Procedures for Virus and Rickettsial Diseases,* American Public Health Association (New York, 1948).
4. Meyer, K. F., B. Eddie, and H. Y. Yanamura, Ornithosis (psittacosis) in pigeons and its relation to human pneumonitis, *Proc. Soc. Exp. Biol. & Med.*, 1942, 49:609.
5. Meyer, K. F., and B. Eddie, Spontaneous ornithosis (psittacosis) in chickens the cause of a human infection, *Proc. Soc. Exp. Biol. & Med.*, 1942, 49:522.
6. Smadel, J. E., M. J. Wall, and A. Gregg, An outbreak of psittacosis in pigeons, involving the production of inclusion bodies, and transfer of the disease to man, *J. Exp. Med.*, 1943, 78:189.
7. Coles, J. D. W. A., Psittacosis in domestic pigeons, Onderstepoort, *J. Vet. Sci.*, 1940, 15:141.
8. Andrewes, C. H., and K. C. Mills, Psittacosis (ornithosis) virus in English pigeons, *Lancet*, 1943, 1:292.
9. Rake, G., *Diagnostic Procedures for Virus and Rickettsial Diseases,* American Public Health Association (New York, 1948).
10. (a) Gönnert, R., Die Bronchopneumonie, eine neue Viruskrankheit der Maus, *Zentralbl. f. Bakt.* (Abt. 1), Orig., 1941, 147:161.

(b) Gönnert, R., Uber ein neues, dem Erreger des Lymphogranuloma inguinale ähnliches Mäusevirus, *Klin. Wchnschr.*, 1941, 20:76.
11. de Burgh, P., A. V. Jackson, and S. F. Williams, Spontaneous infection of laboratory mice with a psittacosis-like organism, *Australian J. Exp. Biol. & Med. Sci.*, 1945, 23:107.
12. Wall, M. J., Isolation of virus of lymphogranuloma venereum from twenty-eight patients; relative value of the use of chick embryos and mice, *J. Immunol.*, 1946, 54:59.
13. Yanamura, H. Y., and K. F. Meyer, Studies on the virus of psittacosis cultivated *in vitro*, *J. Infect. Dis.*, 1941, 68:1.
14. (a) Rake, G., and H. Jones, A toxic factor associated with the agent of lymphogranuloma venereum, *Proc. Soc. Exp. Biol. & Med.*, 1943, 53:86.
(b) Rake, G., and H. Jones, Studies on lymphogranuloma venereum. II. The association of specific toxins with agents of lymphogranuloma-psittacosis group, *J. Exp. Med.*, 1944, 79:463.
15. Hilleman, M. R., Immunological studies on the psittacosis-lymphogranuloma group of viral agents, *J. Infect. Dis.*, 1945, 76:96.
16. Rake, G., M. D. Eaton, and M. F. Shaffer, Similarities and possible relationships among viruses of psittacosis, meningopneumonitis, and lymphogranuloma venereum, *Proc. Soc. Exp. Biol. & Med.*, 1941, 48:528.
17. Eddie, B., and T. Francis, Jr., Occurrence of psittacosis-like infection in domestic and game birds of Michigan, *Proc. Soc. Exp. Biol. & Med.*, 1942, 50:291.
18. Wall, M. J., Complement-fixing antibodies of lymphogranuloma venereum in mice: Their development and response to sulfonamide therapy, *J. Immunol.*, 1947, 55:353.
19. (a) Bedson, S. P., Observations bearing on the antigenic composition of psittacosis virus, *Brit. J. Exp. Path.*, 1936, 17:109.
(b) Bedson, S. P., Observations on the complement-fixation test in psittacosis, *Lancet*, 1937, 2:1477.
20. Smadel, J. E., K. Wertman, and R. L. Reagan, Yolk sac complement fixation antigen for use in psittacosis-lymphogranuloma venereum group of diseases, *Proc. Soc. Exp. Biol. & Med.*, 1943, 54:70.
21. Shaffer, M. F., and G. Rake, Studies on lymphogranuloma venereum: Evaluation of the complement fixation test with Lygranum, *J. Lab. & Clin. Med.*, 1947, 32:1060.
22. Shaffer, M. F., H. Jones, A. W. Grace, D. M. Hamre, and G. Rake, Use of the yolk sac of the developing chicken embryo in the isolation of the agent of lymphogranuloma venereum, *J. Infect. Dis.*, 1944, 75:109.
23. Rake, G., C. M. McKee, and M. F. Shaffer, Agent of lymphogranuloma venereum in the yolk-sac of the developing chick embryo, *Proc. Soc. Exp. Biol. & Med.*, 1940, 43:332.
24. Grace, A. W., G. Rake, and M. F. Shaffer, A new material (Lygranum) for performance of the Frei test for lymphogranuloma venereum, *Proc. Soc. Exp. Biol. & Med.*, 1940, 45:259.

25. Grace, A. W., and F. H. Suskind, Successive transmission of virus of lymphogranuloma inguinale through white mice, *Proc. Soc. Exp. Biol. & Med.*, 1934, 32:71.
26. Frei, W., Eine neue Hautreaktion bei Lymphogranuloma inguinale, *Klin. Wchnschr.*, 1925, 4:2148.
27. (a) Nigg, C., Action of urea and ether on agent and complement-fixing antigen of *Lymphogranuloma venereum*, *Proc. Soc. Exp. Biol. & Med.*, 1942, 49:132.
    (b) Nigg, C., M. R. Hilleman, and B. M. Bowser, Studies on lymphogranuloma venereum complement-fixing antigens. I. Enhancement by phenol or boiling, *J. Immunol.*, 1946, 53:259.
28. Jones, H., G. Rake, and B. Stearns, Studies on lymphogranuloma venereum. III. The action of the sulfonamides on the agent of lymphogranuloma venereum, *J. Infect. Dis.*, 1945, 76:55.
29. Thygeson, P., *Diagnostic Procedures for Virus and Rickettsial Diseases*, American Public Health Association (New York, 1948).
30. Rake, G., M. F. Shaffer, and P. Thygeson, Relationship of agents of trachoma and inclusion conjunctivitis to those of lymphogranuloma-psittacosis group, *Proc. Soc. Exp. Biol. & Med.*, 1942, 49:545.
31. Rice, C. E., Carbohydrate matrix of epithelial-cell inclusion in trachoma, *Am. J. Ophth.*, 1936, 19:1.
32. Pinkerton, H., and V. Moragues, Comparative study of meningopneumonitis virus, psittacosis of pigeon origin, and psittacosis of parrot origin, *J. Exp. Med.*, 1942, 75:575.

Chapter 5

THE DIAGNOSIS OF PRIMARY ATYPICAL PNEUMONIA

By Frank L. Horsfall, Jr., *Hospital of The Rockefeller Institute for Medical Research*

Most workers who have carefully studied patients with primary atypical pneumonia are now inclined to think of the condition as an infectious disease entity. This point of view was supported by the discovery in 1943 that three peculiar and unusual serological phenomena occur during the illness but do not occur, or occur only in exceptional instances, in other infectious diseases. Peterson and co-workers (1), as well as Turner (2), showed that the serum of patients may cause cold agglutination of human group O erythrocytes. Thomas and co-workers (3) showed that serum of patients may give positive complement-fixation reactions with animal-tissue antigens. Thomas and co-workers (4) also demonstrated that serum of patients may cause specific agglutination of a previously unidentified species of nonhemolytic streptococcus, now designated streptococcus MG. These serological reactions served to differentiate the illness from other forms of pneumonia and provided a basis for further study.

Additional evidence in support of the idea that the condition is an infectious disease was provided by the results of transmission experiments in human beings which were carried out by the Commission on Acute Respiratory Diseases (5). These investigators showed that the disease could be induced in approximately one volunteer in four after inoculation of pooled throat washings and sputa into the respiratory tract. The inoculation of bacteria-free filtrates of such specimens also resulted in the development of the illness, and it was concluded that the primary incitant is a filterable agent, presumably a virus. This concept is consistent with various other findings and in accord with ideas regarding the etiology of the condition which have been expressed frequently during recent years. It should be pointed out, however, that in these transmission experiments approximately two volunteers in four developed respiratory infections which could not be called primary atypical pneumonia. Inasmuch as pooled specimens obtained from a number of patients were used as inocula, it is possible that a variety of infectious agents were introduced. If this were the case, it may not be surprising that more than a single clinical syndrome were observed. On the other hand, it may be that but a single filterable agent was present in the inocula and that the different clinical entities seen were caused by the same agent. Recent experiments in human volunteers carried out by the Commission (6) afford some support for the hypothesis that the different clinical syndromes were due to different infectious agents. However, there is still much uncertainty as to whether most, or even the majority, of cases of primary atypical pneumonia are to be attributed to a single infectious agent.

In the case of this disease, in contrast to most of the viral and rickettsial infections which are discussed in this symposium, it appears important to decide what it is we are to discuss rather than to proceed on the assumption that there is unanimous accord on the meaning of the term primary atypical pneumonia. At the present time it seems unwise to attempt to define this condition in terms other than those of a common clinical syndrome which has been recognized and described with increasing frequency and detail during the past decade. It is necessary to rely on the clinical acumen and skill of the numerous workers who have investigated this condition, as well as upon the large body of negative evidence which they have amassed, in order to differentiate this form of pneumonia from others. The usefulness and the limitations of available diagnostic methods will, of necessity, be surveyed against this background. For the purpose of this discussion it will be convenient to make the assumption that the condition is a disease entity, even though unequivocal evidence for this is lacking.

To make a trustworthy diagnosis in primary atypical pneumonia, it is essential to obtain a considerable amount of clinical, X-ray, and laboratory evidence. To establish the diagnosis it is necessary to accumulate all of this evidence and, in addition, to demonstrate that certain serological tests are definitely positive. Unfortunately, this is not an easy task and requires much time. It is only rarely that the diagnosis can be established within a week after the onset, and usually this is not accomplished until the second week. The laboratory procedures which are most useful are the following: (a) bacteriological examination of the sputum and blood; (b) total leucocyte count and leucocyte pattern; (c) cold hemagglutination test; (d) streptococcus MG agglutination test; (e) serological tests with the psittacosis and influenza groups of viruses as well as Q fever rickettsiae.

When, in conjunction with certain clinical findings, there are also the following findings: pulmonary consolidation demonstrable by X-ray, no abnormal bacteriological flora in the respiratory tract, normal leucocyte count and pattern, positive cold hemagglutination test, positive streptococcus MG agglutination test, and negative serological tests with the infectious agents mentioned above, it can be concluded that the diagnosis is primary atypical pneumonia. When, with similar findings, only one of the agglutination tests but not the other is positive, the diagnosis is still on solid ground. It is when both agglutination tests remain persistently negative that difficulties arise and the diagnosis rests on a somewhat insecure basis. It appears now that the number of cases which fail to give positive agglutination tests is at least as large as and is probably larger than the number which show such reactions. This raises a difficulty in accurate diagnosis which has not yet been surmounted.

No signs or symptoms which are pathognomonic have been described. Although there is often a fairly definite clinical syndrome, there are wide variations in the manifestations of the illness. Only five common symptoms have been present in 50 per cent or more of the patients. In order of frequency they are: cough, sputum, headache, malaise, and chilliness. Similarly, only five common physical signs have been present in 50 percent or more of the patients. In analogous order they are: fever, indefinite pulmonary signs, pharyngitis, relative bradycardia, and nasal congestion (7).

The X-ray picture is usually different from that seen in bacterial pneumonias, but it is doubtful that the condition can be identified on X-ray evidence alone. Tuberculosis and psittacosis, for example, may present X-ray findings indistinguishable from those obtained in primary atypical pneumonia.

It is of interest that the disturbance in chloride metabolism which occurs in pneumococcal pneumonia is not found in the disease. Similarly, plasma α-amino-acid levels are within normal limits in primary atypical pneumonia, although they are significantly reduced in bacterial pneumonia (8). Thus, it appears that there may be fundamental differences in the biochemical abnormalities associated with this form of pneumonia as compared to others.

Bacteriological examination of the sputum shows the usual array of microbial species commonly found in the upper respiratory tract of normal persons. Only rarely can type-specific pneumococci be demonstrated directly in sputum, but such microorganisms can be isolated by mouse inoculation from at least two-thirds of the patients. The frequency with which various pneumococcal types are found is similar to their distribution among normal persons. With semiselective media streptococcus MG has been isolated from the sputum of 55 percent of a large series of cases (9). The presence of this microorganism is not an important diagnostic finding because it can be isolated from about 20 percent of cases with other forms of pneumonia and also can be demonstrated in the upper respiratory tract of about 12 percent of normal persons (9). Blood cultures are invariably sterile.

Serological studies have consistently failed to show the development of antibodies against any of the viruses or rickettsiae known to be capable of causing pneumonia in man (10, 11). The agents employed were the following: the influenza group, including strains of A, B, and swine viruses; the psittacosis group of viruses; lymphocytic choriomeningitis virus; Q fever rickettsiae.

The finding that cold hemagglutinins develop during the course of the illness (1, 2) stimulated numerous studies on this phenomenon. Results obtained in over 800 patients diagnosed as primary atypical pneumonia and in over 1,700 patients with other conditions have been published (12). In the former group cold hemagglutinins were demonstrated in 56.7 percent, whereas in the latter group the incidence was only 4.4 percent. The distribution of the maximum cold hemagglutination titers observed in three series of patients (13, 14, 15) is shown in Table 1. These patients were largely selected, and therefore the results probably do not represent what would be obtained with unselected cases. It is evident that there are wide variations in the titers found and that 50 percent of these cases failed to develop titers higher than 1:40. Even though low concentrations of human group O erythrocytes are employed to increase the sensitivity of the test—0.2 percent red cells were used in the second series—a large proportion

Table 1

COLD HEMAGGLUTINATION TITERS IN PRIMARY ATYPICAL PNEUMONIA

Reference	No. of Patients Studied	Maximum Titer No. of Patients Showing—									
		0	10	20	40	80	160	320	640	1280	2560 or >
13	200	45	9	9	23	23	28	27	14	14	8
14	93	42	8	7	7	5	4	4	7	3	6
15	74	12	2	15	9	10	9	7	6	3	1
Total	367	99	19	31	39	38	41	38	27	20	15
Percent	100	27	5	8	11	10	11	10	7	5	4

of cases fail to develop significant titers. Most workers now employ 1 or 2 percent red-cell suspensions and hold the serum-erythrocyte mixtures at 4°C. overnight before making readings. Warming the mixtures at 37°C. for one hour causes the reaction to disappear; subsequent cooling causes it to reappear. When blood is obtained for cold hemagglutination tests, it is important that the serum be separated before the specimen is refrigerated. If this precaution is not taken, much or all of the cold agglutinin may be discarded with the clotted cells. Cold agglutinins appear to be relatively unstable and tend to disappear during prolonged storage. However, their titer is unaffected by heating sera at 56°C. for thirty minutes.

Of more significance than the finding of a fairly high titer of cold agglutinins is the demonstration of a significant increase in titer during the course of the illness. To accomplish this, it is necessary to examine a number of specimens of serum obtained at various times— for example, at weekly intervals—after the onset. Finland and co-workers (16) showed that a definite increase in titer occurred only in exceptional instances in conditions other than primary atypical pneumonia. They also demonstrated that maximum titers are usually found two to three weeks after onset and that titers progressively decline during the first and second months after the illness. It has been found that both the incidence of cold agglutinins and the height of the maximum titer are related to the severity of the illness as judged by either the height or the duration of fever (13). The more severe the attack, the more likely are cold agglutinins to develop and the higher is the titer. These findings do not provide support for the hypothesis (6) that attacks which are associated with cold agglutinins may be of different etiology from those in which such agglutinins fail to appear.

The isolation of streptococcus MG from the lung tissues of six fatal cases and the demonstration that specific antibodies against this microorganism often develop during the course of the illness stimulated a number of studies. Results of streptococcus MG agglutination tests with serum from more than 660 patients with primary atypical pneumonia and more than 560 patients with other diseases have been published (12). Positive tests were obtained in 44 percent of the former series and in 4 percent of the latter. However, it should be pointed out that a fourfold or greater increase in agglutination titer against streptococcus MG has almost never been encountered except in primary atypical pneumonia. The distribution of the maximum titers obtained in three large series of cases (9, 17, 18) is shown in Table 2. The third series is composed entirely of cases which showed

TABLE 2

STREPTOCOCCUS MG AGGLUTINATION TITERS IN PRIMARY ATYPICAL PNEUMONIA

Reference	No. of Patients Studied	Maximum Titer No. of Patients Showing—						
		0	10	20	40	80	160	320 or >
9	193	63	54	35	19	16	4	2
17	156	83	31	31	10	0	1	0
18	78	7	11	23	15	19	3	0
Total	427	153	96	89	44	35	8	2
Percent	100	36	22	21	10	8	2	0.5

positive cold agglutination tests; cases in the other two series were not selected on this basis. It will be seen that the maximum titers found vary considerably, but are not strikingly high in any instance. Only about 2.5 percent of cases developed titers of 1:160 or higher, and no fewer than 58 percent failed to show titers higher than 1:10. It may be pertinent to recall that in pneumococcal pneumonia, serum agglutination titers against the homologous type bacterium are of a similar low order.

In carrying out agglutination tests with streptococcus MG, a suspension of heat-killed and washed bacteria is employed (9). The turbidity is carefully standardized, preferably by photoelectric means, because the titers obtained are inversely related to the concentration of microorganisms used. Suspensions which are properly prepared remain stable and give reproducible results for many months if stored at 4°C. Serum is not heated at 56°C. before the test because this may sometimes reduce the titer. Serum-streptococcal suspension mixtures are best held for twelve to eighteen hours at room temperature before the results are read. Antibodies against the microorganism are not adsorbed by red blood cells in the cold, and the precautions mentioned in connection with refrigerating blood before cold agglutination tests do not apply when streptococcus MG agglutination tests are to be performed.

The demonstration of a definite increase in titer during or shortly after the illness is of much greater diagnostic significance than the finding of agglutinins against the bacterium in a single specimen of serum. As with tests for cold agglutinins, it is desirable that serum be obtained at weekly intervals for streptococcus MG agglutination tests. The incidence of positive tests increases during the first four to five weeks after onset and thereafter decreases gradually (10). In most instances antibodies make their first appearance following defervescence of fever. Maximum titers are usually present by the fourth week.

Curnen and co-workers (10) showed that both the incidence of antibodies against the microorganism and the height of the maximum agglutination titer were directly related to the duration of the illness. The duration of fever, signs of pneumonia, X-ray evidence of pneumonia, and the period of hospitalization were in each instance correlated with the maximum titer of agglutinins against streptococcus MG. Thus, it appears that the incidence of both cold agglutinins and streptococcal agglutinins is directly proportional to the severity or duration of the illness. Present evidence suggests that neither test is very sensitive and that the threshold for definitely positive reactions with either test may be fairly high. It seems reasonable to assume that quantitative factors relating to the degree of stimulation provided by the infection rather than qualitative factors relating to possible differences in cause may be decisive in determining the development of positive serological reactions.

As is shown in Table 3, there is not a very close correlation between

TABLE 3

CORRELATION OF STREPTOCOCCUS MG AND COLD HEMAGGLUTINATION REACTIONS IN PRIMARY ATYPICAL PNEUMONIA (9, 17, 18)

COLD HEM-AGGLUTINATION Number of Cases	STREPTOCOCCUS MG AGGLUTINATION Number of Cases		TOTAL Number of Cases
	POSITIVE	NEGATIVE	
Positive	120	33	153
Negative	22	61	83
Total	142	94	236
Percentage of Cases	Percentage of Cases		Percentage of Cases
	POSITIVE	NEGATIVE	
Positive	51	14	65
Negative	9	26	35
Total	60	40	100

cold agglutination and streptococcus MG agglutination reactions. These results were obtained in three independent series of cases (9, 17, 18). It will be noted that one reaction was positive and the other negative in no fewer than 23 percent of patients. This suggests that the two reactions are not caused by the same component in serum. In this connection it is of interest that Thomas and co-workers (9) demonstrated by means of cross-absorption tests, that either cold agglutinins or agglutinins against streptococcus MG could be removed selectively from convalescent serum without affecting the other reaction.

Not only are agglutinins against the streptococcus demonstrable with serum from patients, but also precipitins directed against the purified capsular polysaccharide of the microorganism and capsular swelling antibodies have been found (9). Moreover, by means of induced nonencapsulated R variants it has been shown that antibodies directed against somatic antigens of the bacterium also develop during the course of the illness (9). In the light of these findings it is difficult to escape the conclusion that a specific immunological response occurs and that the stimulus responsible is streptococcus MG itself.

If the infectious agent responsible for primary atypical pneumonia were readily transmissible to laboratory animals, it is probable that highly specific diagnostic procedures could be developed, as has been

TABLE 4

NEUTRALIZATION TESTS WITH E.M.H. VIRUS (19) AND SERUM FROM PATIENTS WITH PRIMARY ATYPICAL PNEUMONIA

Serum	Dil.	No. of Hamsters	Pulmonary Lesions			Percentage	
			\multicolumn{3}{c}{No. of Hamsters Having}		
			0	±	+ or >	±	+ or >
Normal animal (control)	1:4	124	44	16	64	13	52
Acute PAP (8 cases; 4–9 days)	1:4	55	28	6	21	11	38
	1:16	49	23	9	17	18	35
	1:64	15	10	2	3	13	20
Conval. PAP (8 cases; 20–44 days)	1:4	55	46	7	2	13	4
	1:16	45	39	3	3	7	7
	1:64	50	44	2	4	4	8

accomplished already with most of the infectious diseases under consideration in this symposium. Numerous efforts to recover an infectious agent by means of animal inoculation have led to confusing and conflicting results. At least five apparently different agents, each of which may be a virus, have been put forward as possible etiological factors during the past nine years (12). All of the agents which have been claimed to be transmissible to animals possessed properties which made it difficult to devise decisive experiments; each had very low pathogenicity for the animal species employed.

Eaton and co-workers (19) have presented the most impressive evidence so far obtained for the recovery of a virus from patients. Through the courtesy of Dr. Eaton, we were able to obtain strains of this virus, as well as immune serum against it, and carried out a series of investigations with the agent. The results of neutralization tests with the virus and serum from patients are presented in summary form in Table 4. The technical procedures described by the workers who recovered the agent were followed to the letter. Acute-phase and convalescent-serum specimens from eight patients studied in the Hospital of The Rockefeller Institute were employed individually. Each of the patients developed antibodies against streptococcus MG, and all tested also developed cold agglutinins. It is evident that the incidence of pulmonary lesions in hamsters inoculated intranasally with convalescent serum-virus mixtures was lower than that obtained in animals given acute-phase serum-virus mixtures. These results are essentially similar to those described by Eaton and his associates (20).

The results of neutralization tests with the virus and serum of rabbits or hamsters immunized with various antigens are shown in Table 5. It will be noted that not only the homologous antiserum but also antisera prepared against tissue suspensions containing either influenza viruses or PVM, as well as antiserum against normal chick-embryo tissue itself, caused a reduction in the incidence of pulmonary lesions. In contrast, the serum of animals recovered from infection with either influenza viruses or PVM, as well as antiserum against streptococcus MG, caused no similar reduction in the incidence of such lesions. Because the former group of antisera contained antibodies reactive with normal embryo material, whereas the latter group did not, it appeared possible that the occurrence of antigen-antibody reactions not specifically related to the virus might lead to apparent neutraliza-

TABLE 5

NEUTRALIZATION TESTS WITH E.M.H. VIRUS AND SERUM FROM IMMUNE ANIMALS

Serum	Dil.	No. of Hamsters	Pulmonary Lesions				
			No. of Hamsters with—			Percentage	
			0	±	+ or >	±	+ or >
Normal animal (control)	1:4	124	44	16	64	13	52
Anti-E.M.H. virus (Embr.)	1:4	20	14	4	2	20	10
	1:16	10	9	1	0	10	0
Anti-norm. Embr.	1:4	20	11	1	3	5	15
Anti-infl. virus (Embr.)	1:4	10	9	0	1	0	10
Anti-PVM (M. lung)	1:4	8	6	0	2	0	25
Total		38	26	1	6	3	16
Anti-strep. MG	1:4	10	4	3	3	30	30
Conval. infl. virus	1:4	10	4	1	5	10	50
Conval. PVM	1:4	5	2	1	2	20	40
Total		25	10	5	10	20	40

TABLE 6

NEUTRALIZATION TESTS WITH ABSORBED PAP SERUM AND E.M.H. VIRUS

Serum	Absorbed with—	Dil.	No. of Hamsters	Pulmonary Lesions			Percentage	
				No. of Hamsters with—				
				0	±	+ or >	±	+ or >
Acute PAP (2 cases; 4–6 days)	O (control)	1:4	10	5	2	3	20	30
		1:16	10	6	0	4	0	40
	Strep. MG.	1:4	10	4	4	2	40	20
		1:16	10	7	1	2	10	20
	Norm. M. lung	1:4	10	4	5	1	50	10
		1:16	10	3	4	3	40	30
Conval. PAP (2 cases; 29–44 days)	O (control)	1:4	10	9	1	0	10	0
		1:16	10	8	0	2	0	20
	Strep. MG.	1:4	10	6	2	2	20	20
		1:16	10	4	3	3	30	30
	Norm. M. lung	1:4	10	6	2	2	20	20
		1:16	10	6	2	2	20	20

tion of the agent. It should be pointed out that owing to the low pathogenicity of the virus, it was necessary to use suspensions containing a considerable amount of infected embryo material in the neutralization tests.

It will be recalled that there is evidence indicating that convalescent serum from patients may contain a component which reacts with antigens present in normal animal tissues (3). Because of the possibility mentioned above, absorption experiments were carried out to determine the effect of removal of this component from human convalescent serum. In Table 6 are shown the results of neutralization tests with the virus and serum of two patients after the serum specimens had been absorbed either with streptococcus MG or with normal mouse lung tissue. Both patients developed antibodies against the streptococcus and were included in the group of eight patients mentioned previously. It will be seen that, although the unabsorbed convalescent sera caused a reduction in the incidence of pulmonary lesions in hamsters, neither the specimens absorbed with streptococcus MG nor those absorbed with normal mouse-lung tissue caused a similar reduction. These results appear to support the hypothesis that antigen-antibody reactions unrelated to the virus may cause apparent neutralization of the agent. Moreover, they raise important questions as to the significance of the results of neutralization tests with convalescent serum obtained from patients with this illness.

In the light of these findings it appears doubtful that unequivocal evidence for the development of specific antibodies against a virus has been obtained as yet in primary atypical pneumonia. At the present time the chief laboratory procedures which are useful in establishing a diagnosis are cold hemagglutination and streptococcus MG agglutination tests. Unfortunately, the limitations of both tests leave much to be desired.

REFERENCES

1. Peterson, O. L., T. H. Ham, and M. Finland, Cold agglutinins (autohemagglutinins) in primary atypical pneumonias, *Science*, 1943, 97:167.
2. Turner, J. C., Development of cold-agglutinins in atypical pneumonia, *Nature*, 1943, 151:419.
3. Thomas, L., *et al.*, Complement fixation with dissimilar antigens in primary atypical pneumonia, *Proc. Soc. Exp. Biol. & Med.*, 1943, 52:121.

4. Thomas, L., et al., Serological reactions with an indifferent streptococcus in primary atypical pneumonia, *Science*, 1943, 98:566.
5. Commission on Acute Respiratory Diseases, The transmission of primary atypical pneumonia to human volunteers, *Bull. Johns Hopkins Hosp.*, 1946, 79:97.
6. Commission on Acute Respiratory Diseases, Experimental transmission of minor respiratory illness to human volunteers by filter-passing agents, I: Demonstration of two types of illness characterized by long and short incubation periods and different clinical features; II: Immunity on reinoculation with agents from the two types of minor respiratory illness and from primary atypical pneumonia, *J. Clin. Invest.*, 1947, 26:957, 974.
7. Horsfall, F. L., Jr., Primary atypical pneumonia and influenza—diagnosis, prevention, treatment, *Bull. N. Y. Acad. Med.*, 1948, 24:431.
8. Emerson, K., Jr., et al., Chloride metabolism and plasma amino acid levels in primary atypical pneumonia, *J. Clin. Invest.*, 1943, 22:695.
9. Thomas, L., et al., Studies on primary atypical pneumonia, II: Observations concerning the relationship of a non-hemolytic streptococcus to the disease, *J. Clin. Invest.*, 1945, 24:227.
10. Curnen, E. C., et al., Studies on primary atypical pneumonia, I: Clinical features and results of laboratory investigations, *J. Clin. Invest.*, 1945, 24:209.
11. Dingle, J. H., et al., Primary atypical pneumonia, etiology unknown, *War Med.*, 1943, 3:223.
12. Horsfall, F. L., Jr., Primary atypical pneumonia, *Ann. Int. Med.*, 1947, 27:275.
13. Finland, M., et al., Cold agglutinins, II: Cold isohemagglutinins in primary atypical pneumonia of unknown etiology with a note on the occurrence of hemolytic anemia in these cases, *J. Clin. Invest.*, 1945, 24:458.
14. Commission on Acute Respiratory Diseases, Cold hemagglutinins in primary atypical pneumonia and other respiratory infections, *Am. J. Med. Sci.*, 1944, 208:742.
15. Meiklejohn, G., The cold agglutination test in the diagnosis of primary atypical pneumonia, *Proc. Soc. Exp. Biol. & Med.*, 1943, 54:181.
16. Finland, M., et al., Cold agglutinins, I: Occurrence of cold isohemagglutinins in various conditions, *J. Clin. Invest.*, 1945, 24:451.
17. Meiklejohn, G., and V. L. Hanford, Agglutination tests with streptococcus No. 344 in primary atypical pneumonia, *Proc. Soc. Exp. Biol. & Med.*, 1944, 57:356.
18. Finland, M., et al., Cold agglutinins, VI: Agglutinins for an indifferent streptococcus in primary atypical pneumonia and in other conditions and their relation to cold isohemagglutinins, *J. Clin. Invest.*, 1945, 24:497.
19. Eaton, M. D., et al., Studies on the etiology of primary atypical pneu-

monia; a filterable agent transmissible to cotton rats, hamsters and chick embryos, *J. Exp. Med.*, 1944, 79:649.
20. Eaton, M. D., *et al.*, Studies on the etiology of primary atypical pneumonia, III: Specific neutralization of the virus by human serum, *J. Exp. Med.*, 1945, 82:329.

Chapter 6

THE DIAGNOSIS OF NEUROTROPIC VIRUS INFECTIONS, INCLUDING THE VIRAL ENCEPHALITIDES, LYMPHOCYTIC CHORIOMENINGITIS, AND POLIOMYELITIS

By JORDI CASALS AND PETER K. OLITSKY, *The Rockefeller Institute for Medical Research*

FOR THE PRESENT, the diagnosis of neurotropic virus infections, including the viral encephalitides, lymphocytic choriomeningitis and poliomyelitis, depends on the clinical picture; on the isolation and identification of the virus; on the formation of the specific antibody of virus neutralization and of complement fixation; for purposes of differential diagnosis, on changes in the blood picture and the cerebrospinal fluid; finally, post-mortem, on the pathological picture. Other modern laboratory procedures, such as electroencephalography, direct visualization of virus by the electron microscope, and serological tests of agglutination, cold agglutination, or hemagglutination, are not as yet applicable to the diagnosis of these diseases.

In this discussion, we shall dwell upon the laboratory means of diagnosis and stress the limitations and reservations of such means for identifying the specific etiological agent of the malady in question.

THE HUMAN VIRAL ENCEPHALITIDES INCLUDING LYMPHOCYTIC CHORIOMENINGITIS

The arthropod-borne types. Of the viral encephalitides the largest group is included in the arthropod-borne encephalitides, so named by Hammon and Reeves: Western equine, Eastern equine, Venezuelan equine, St. Louis, Japanese B (which may also be the prototype of Australian X), Russian Far East (tick-borne or spring-summer) encephalitides and probably louping-ill. In nature, the last-mentioned illness attacks sheep, especially in Scotland, North England, and perhaps Western Russia; the vector is a sheep tick. Certain infections have been met in persons in contact with the virus during laboratory work, as is shown by Rivers and Schwentker (1). Recently, observers have reported the disease in human beings in White Russia, although Scottish and English contacts have thus far not been affected by clinically demonstrable louping-ill. The disease is described here because its virus has a close serological relationship to the Russian Far East encephalitis, as was demonstrated by Casals (2).

The outstanding points of similarity of one member of the group of arthropod-borne encephalitides to another are the clinical and pathological pictures, for no practical classification based on these features can be made, except for certain additional histopathological changes in the cerebellum in Japanese B encephalitis. Here the Purkinje cells are largely degenerated and often completely destroyed, and their destruction leaves empty gaps or spaces in the tissue. In this respect the changes are similar to those found in nature and in the experimental disease in louping-ill. Other points of similarity are that the viruses of this group of maladies are mostly of the same size, about 20-30 millimicrons in diameter; they are all arthropod-borne and pathogenic for albino mice, especially the Swiss W strain, and for chick embryos, growing actively in the tissues of mice and embryos to yield titers of 10^{-7} to 10^{-9}, even rarely 10^{-10}. Three of the group, Western and Eastern equine and St. Louis viruses, have been found to prevail at the same time in the same areas, and the Western and St. Louis types have been said to have the same species of vector and of reservoir (Hammon and colleagues) (3). In view of these and other considerations, several workers, including the writers, have postulated a single common ancestor of this group. However this may be, the viruses are not identical; in one way or another distinctive features can be brought to the surface.

The clinical and pathological pictures are, then, indicative only of an encephalitis; the differentiation of the various members into specific types is possible only through laboratory investigations which combine the isolation and identification of the virus and serological and immunological procedures.

For isolation of the virus, the most suitable material is the tissue of the central nervous system. This applies to all of the arthropod-borne encephalitides, including the Venezuelan equine encephalitis as it occurs in nature. In the case of the latter disease as it arises in the nonarthropod-borne, nonfatal case, that is, in those exposed to the virus in laboratory work, nasopharyngeal washings or blood is the source of virus. The materials are inoculated intracerebrally in mice, preferably the Swiss strain. The identification of a recovered virus is then achieved by means of serological tests, either neutralization or complement-fixation, or both: (a) prepared standard antisera are tested against the virus; (b) antiserum derived from animals immunized to the recovered virus is tested for antibody against standard stock viruses; (c) immunity to the virus is sought for in animals vaccinated with standard strains of virus; and finally, (d) the latter can be performed also in a reverse manner, that is, vaccination first of animals with the virus in question and the test of their immunity made with standard viruses. In practice, however, the first procedure, namely, neutralization and/or complement fixation by means of the recovered virus and prepared standard antisera can suffice; it usually does.

Tests are also made on the patient's serum specifically for the development of neutralizing or protective, and complement-fixing antibody. For appraisal of results it should be taken into consideration that a close serological relationship exists between louping-ill and Russian Far East viruses; that serological overlapping is found among the Japanese B, St. Louis, and West Nile viruses; and that a certain small degree of crossing in complement fixation by Eastern and Western equine viruses is sometimes noted. These difficulties in appraisal can be resolved, however, by observation of the strength of the reactions, since the homologous reactions are, as a rule, stronger than the heterologous, and, for differentiation of louping-ill from the Russian virus, by the use of the intracerebral immunity test in mice, which is more specific than serological procedures.

An interesting problem is the meaning of the overlapping of serological reactions within the group of arthropod-borne encephalitides. It may be a reflection of the crudity of the tests as carried out—a lack of fineness to delineate specific responses—or possibly it represents an antigenic factor common to members of this group. If a new encephalitic strain which is more antigenically inclusive were found, it would add evidence for the latter view (4).

Another pitfall in interpretation of results of serological tests is the tendency of these viruses to induce clinically inapparent or abortive infections in endemic and epidemic areas. Thus, a varying number of normal-appearing persons who have no recollection of a definite encephalitic disease can be found to possess specific antibody. To overcome this obstacle, the test is carried out with serum obtained from the patient at the earliest stage of his malady as well as with another one or two serum specimens collected from one to three or even more weeks later, during convalescence; sometimes less than one week of convalescence suffices (5, 6). If the first specimen is negative and the later ones show an upsurge of antibody content, or a level of antibody definitely higher than that exhibited by the first serum, then a positive diagnosis can be made. If the early sample is negative and the later ones are also negative, the diagnosis is either negative or made cautiously, since a still later sample may be positive. If, on the other hand, the early sample has an antibody content equal to or higher than the later ones the test may be unsuitable.

Another difficulty in the diagnostic procedures lies in the fact that much time is often needed, up to two or three weeks, before a definite result is known. In skillful hands, in a well-organized laboratory, and in a situation where the precise type of virus is predictable, the time can be shortened to a few days, instead of weeks, as has been demonstrated by Sabin and his colleagues (6) for Japanese B encephalitis in Korea. Even though the results of the tests as they are generally carried out may be known to the individual—the subject of the tests—at a time when they are of little use to him, this information is of the greatest value to the epidemiologist and the clinician in support of their knowledge of the specific type of encephalitis that is prevalent.

Other examinations carried out in the laboratory in cases of arthropod-borne encephalitides relate to changes in the blood count and in the cerebrospinal-fluid pictures. The usual reaction in all forms is one of a moderate degree of leucocytosis (10,000–25,000 cells), ordinarily of the polymorphonuclear type. The cerebrospinal fluid exhibits, as a rule, varying degrees of pleocytosis of mononuclear type (polymorphonuclear cells can, however, predominate early), varying degrees of increase in protein, and a normal amount of sugar. These changes are, of course, nonspecific, but they may be of value for differential diagnosis of the viral encephalitides from other conditions.

Types transmitted by direct contact with lower animals. The maladies of this group are: infections with B virus, swineherd's disease, encephalomyocarditis, Mengo encephalomyelitis, lymphocytic choriomeningitis, and rabies, which is discussed in another paper of this series. The other diseases either have occurred thus far rarely, or were generally nonfatal, with the exception of B virus infection, so that the diagnosis rests chiefly on a history of exposure to the virus, the clinical picture, and only in certain instances on laboratory procedures.

Infection with *Sabin's B virus* of monkeys led, in the only case thoroughly studied, to a fatal, acute, ascending myelitis associated with focal necrosis of the internal organs. Two others succumbed to the bites of normal-seeming monkeys, which can harbor the virus in the saliva. The virus produces in experimental animals multinucleated giant cells and intranuclear inclusion bodies of the herpetic type. It has properties in common with the viruses of herpes simplex and pseudorabies; they are serologically related in the manner noted among certain members of the arthropod-borne group of encephalitides. The crossing is not at high levels; the homologous reactions are stronger than the heterologous. When normal human serum shows neutralizing antibody for herpes simplex virus it also may react with B virus, as Burnet (7) has shown; he states that the B virus is a more inclusive antigen. Normal-appearing monkeys reveal to a greater or lesser degree, depending on the stock, serum neutralizing antibody for B virus. Other points of differentiation of this virus from that of herpes simplex and pseudorabies, as stated by Sabin (8), are that the virus of pseudorabies is more pathogenic than the B virus for guinea pigs and mice; both (but not the virus of herpes simplex) are pathogenic for Rhesus monkeys.

It is not yet certain whether *swineherd's disease*, as it occurs in swine and man, is a leptospirosis. Outside of Switzerland this characteristic, nonfatal illness is not associated with leptospiral antibody (Lépine), and it is considered as having a viral etiology. The diagnosis is made by history of exposure to affected swine, by a typical clinical syndrome, and by development of specific virus-neutralizing antibody.

Encephalomyocarditis, a spontaneous disease of apes, is included in this discussion because recently Smadel and Warren (9) described an epidemic among military personnel in Manila, who showed a febrile illness with concomitant headache, coma, stiff neck, or positive Kernig sign, with leucopenia, lymphocytosis, and with pleocytosis of lymphocytic type in the cerebrospinal fluid. In the three cases studied, specific neutralizing antibody developed increasingly in convalescence. Although the virus was not recovered, the inference is that the etiologic agent could be regarded as a virus closely related to that of encephalomyocarditis.

Mengo encephalomyelitis is a newly discovered virus infection of man; the first and only case thus far encountered arose in the Mengo district of Uganda, Africa. A similar virus was recovered from a monkey kept then in the laboratory and from indigenous mosquitoes. Specific neutralizing antibody was found not only in the recovered individual but also in certain other human beings offering no definite history of a clinical attack. A description of this virus will be given in forthcoming papers by G. W. A. Dick; for the present, the interest in this agent lies in its close serological relationship with the viruses of encephalomyocarditis, the MM and the SK viruses (*v. infra*), and the probability of its wide dissemination over the world (G. W. A. Dick, personal communication).

The virus of *lymphocytic choriomeningitis* (LCM) is found in nature in wild mice and is now believed to be transmitted to man by some vector still unknown. Since the virus can be found in rodent urine, nasal secretions, feces, and semen, these materials may have an epidemiological bearing on the dissemination of the disease. This virus may also interfere with the work of the laboratory, since it may spread among normal stock mice and so obfuscate interpretation of results. The clinical picture of the disease in man is protean. As it often resembles "grippe" or mild influenza, however, diagnosis based only on symptoms or signs is difficult, even though the cerebrospinal fluid shows lymphocytic pleocytosis of an unusually high degree. The illness, with rarest exceptions, is nonfatal, and the pathological picture remains ordinarily obscure. The diagnosis, therefore, rests on isolation of the virus and on specific antibody demonstration. For the isolation of the virus, cerebrospinal fluid and blood prove to be the best sources; virus can easily be recovered by inoculation of these fluids into guinea pigs and mice.

Since complement-fixing and neutralizing antibodies appear during convalescence, their detection confirms the diagnosis. The serological reactions in this malady are unlike those of other encephalitides in many respects. Complement fixation is positive sooner than neutralization, appearing first about one to three weeks after onset of illness. Neutralizing antibody may be first noted after six to ten weeks; in the case cited by Florman (10) it was first detected between the seventy-second and the one hundred and thirtieth day. Since persons who appear to be normal may harbor these antibodies, the serological tests should be performed on paired samples, the second taken after a sufficient time has elapsed, as was described for the arthropod-borne encephalitides.

Smadel and colleagues (11) showed that specific complement-fixing antibody for a soluble antigen develops in LCM infection; this antigen is present in large amount in the spleen and other organs in the experimental disease. The splenic tissue antigen, as used by Smadel, by Lépine and co-workers, and by others, is stable, specific, and satisfactory, but in Bedson's hands (12) it yielded only negative results. Bedson warns that freshly prepared antigen may be nonspecific; the tissue should therefore be aged for two or three weeks before use. Casals has found, on the other hand, that mouse-brain antigens are unsatisfactory. However this may be, the point should be stressed that although neutralizing antibody may persist for at least three years, complement-fixing antibody begins to wane or to disappear three to six weeks after the onset of illness.

Finally, Shwartzman (13) has shown that in infected animals, the virus is firmly adherent to the red blood corpuscles. No practical application for diagnosis has yet been made of this finding.

Pseudolymphocytic choriomeningitis is in a class by itself at present because only two instances are recorded, and little is known about the virus and methods of diagnosis. The two cases were clinically designated as acute aseptic meningitis, and the diagnosis was made by isolation of the virus after intracerebral inoculation of spinal fluid into mice. The virus was shown to be distinct from that of lymphocytic choriomeningitis in pathogenicity for laboratory animals, in size, and in serological and immunological reactions.

Encephalitis produced by viruses ordinarily nonencephalitogenic. The encephalitides that arise during the course of an infection by a virus that is usually nonencephalitogenic are those caused by the viruses of herpes simplex, lymphogranuloma venereum, mumps, measles, dengue, and infectious mononucleosis (probably a viral infection). A critical diagnostic point is the differentiation of such conditions from the so-called postinfection encephalitides—those arising after vaccinia, measles, influenza, and other primary viral illnesses. In encephalitis occurring during a primary viral attack, the causal virus is still active and may be recovered while the encephalitic process still goes on; but in the postinfection encephalitides, the primary virus has dropped into the background or has disappeared and is not recoverable. The pathological picture of the postinfection condition reveals in all types characteristic perivascular demyelination and productive inflammation, irrespective of the primary virus involved, whereas in the encephalitides arising during a direct viral attack, the pathological changes are those induced by that virus. The other point in the diagnosis of a viral encephalitis is that a specific diagnosis can be made only by isolation and identification of the virus from the nervous tissue, the cerebrospinal fluid, or other sources, or by demonstration of a specific viral antibody that increases with time after the onset of illness. While there are, as yet, no established laboratory procedures for determining the type of encephalitis, as in measles and infectious mononucleosis, the diagnosis is inferred on clinical bases, including examination of the blood and of the spinal fluid for cellular and chemical changes.

In *herpes simplex encephalitis*, the virus is isolated from the central nervous system, and the pathological picture exhibits the characteristic lesions containing the herpetic type of intranuclear inclusion bodies. In nonfatal cases the diagnosis becomes extremely difficult because the virus can readily be recovered from nonnervous tissues in nonencephalitic, herpetic infections, such as labial herpes or herpetic stomatitis, and specific neutralizing antibody can be found in the majority of normal-appearing adult human beings.

In encephalitis caused by the virus of *lymphogranuloma venereum*, the active agent is recoverable from the cerebrospinal fluid in nonfatal infection. The diagnosis can be complemented by determination of the nature of the local lesion, aided by demonstration of development of specific serum neutralizing and complement-fixing antibody or by use of the Frei skin test. The serological reactions should be expertly assayed because this virus may show crossing with the etiological agents of the psittacosis-trachoma-pneumonitis group of maladies.

The infection of the nervous system with *mumps* virus can take the form of meningitis, encephalitis, or, as it is usually designated, meningo-encephalitis. The nervous form may or may not be associated with involvement of the parotid gland. In view of recent refinements in diagnosis, it is now recognized as a common occurrence in mumps infection. The diagnosis is made by isolation of the mumps virus from the blood, cerebrospinal fluid, and saliva, which, according to Beveridge et al., (14) can be directly inoculated into developing chick embryos. Another aid in diagnosis, developed by Enders (15), is the demonstration of the progressive increase of complement-fixing antibody in serum during convalescence; this is especially valuable in cases that show no apparent parotitis. Enders (16) has also developed a skin test of local sensitivity to mumps virus, which can be helpful in epidemiological studies. Finally, an unusually marked spinal-fluid lymphocytic pleocytosis is observed during the acute phase of the illness.

A steadily increasing number of reports reveal that in different epidemics in various parts of the world individuals ill with *dengue* exhibit meningeal or encephalitic signs associated with significant changes in the spinal fluid. The diagnosis of infection with the virus of dengue is described in another paper of this series.

Viruses encephalitogenic in experimental animals but as yet not found to cause encephalitis in man. Two neurotropic viruses have recently been discovered in Africa which were isolated from the blood of patients ill with nonfatal febrile affections not apparently of encephalitic type; they are the West Nile and Bwamba fever viruses. The diagnosis of the maladies they induce is made by isolation of the virus from the blood and its identification, and demonstration of a progressive development of specific neutralizing antibody in convalescence.

Viruses encephalitogenic in experimental animals but as yet not found to cause any apparent illness in man. Of these viruses, two were discovered in Africa—the Semliki Forest and the Bunyamwera; four in South America—the Ilhéus and the Colombian Anopheles A, Anopheles B, and the Wyeomyia; and one in North America—the Hammon-Reeves California. All have been recovered from mosquitoes trapped in the field. With the exception of the three Colombian strains, they have the capacity to induce specific neutralizing antibody in human beings, that is, to cause clinically unrecognizable infections.[1]

[1] Recently Hammon and Reeves (unpublished) found a single case, an infant having a severe clinical encephalitis probably of the California virus type; the diagnosis was based on the development of specific antibody during the infection.

These two groups of viruses encephalitogenic in experimental animals and the groups that follow are included in this discussion because they sometimes come into view for differential diagnosis of the established forms of the viral encephalitides.

Neurological maladies having possible viral etiology but no infective agent as yet identified. Among these illnesses are von Economo's disease, herpes zoster, and infectious polyneuritis.

Von Economo's disease, or encephalitis lethargica, prevailed widely over the world from 1915 to 1926; thereafter it subsided and became rare. The etiological agent has not been isolated. The diagnosis can therefore only be inferred on clinical, pathological, and epidemiological grounds, and on laboratory tests that reveal no virus or specific antibodies.

Herpes zoster is considered as possibly having a virus etiology on the grounds that it is reported to be transmissible from man to man, the only susceptible species thus far known; that the illness is followed by immunity; and that the cutaneous lesions contain a viral type of intranuclear inclusions. No virus, however, has been recovered. In certain rare instances, encephalitis has developed during the zoster attack. The diagnosis is made on clinical and pathological pictures and on failure to isolate a familiar virus, especially that of herpes simplex, from the vesicular contents during life or from the central or peripheral nervous tissues after death.

Infectious polyneuritis, or the Guillain-Barré syndrome, has been suspected of being a viral disease, but no infective agent has, as yet, been identified with it. The diagnosis is arrived at chiefly on clinical manifestations of involvement of the peripheral spinal and cranial nerves, which may occur after infections by known or unknown agents or, in some cases, arise spontaneously. The syndrome exhibits a markedly increased amount of protein in the cerebrospinal fluid in the absence of pleocytosis, the so-called protein-cytological dissociation. The histopathological changes in the nerves are swelling and beading of the myelin, and fragmentation and dissolution of the axons; those in the neurons of ganglia and the cord are degenerative and chromatolytic lesions simulating those that follow axonal injury.

Encephalitides of suggested but not proved viral etiology. In this class are found acute primary hemorrhagic encephalitis, acute disseminated encephalomyelitis, chronic multiple sclerosis, and the postinfection encephalitides. In the first three, Russian workers (17) have reported the isolation of a virus from the blood or the spinal fluid or both. Until these findings are confirmed, the diagnosis is made on clinical grounds and on pathological changes, especially the characteristic perivascular demyelination.

Still unknown is the causal agent of the large group of postinfection or postvaccinal or demyelinating encephalitides that follow (a) infection with viruses such as measles, influenza, mumps, varicella, vaccinia, variola, and others, or (b) immunization against rabies or smallpox. The diagnosis is arrived at by a history of a preceding viral infection or immunization, usually within two weeks, by the clinical syndrome, and by failure to recover the primary viral agent. Specifically, the diagnosis is confirmed by detection of characteristic perivascular demyelination. As has been mentioned, care should be taken not to confuse the encephalitides that arise during viral diseases (as, for example, mumps meningo-encephalitis) with the demyelinating maladies that follow the viral infections and do not show changes induced by the primary viruses (as, for example, postmumps encephalitis).

POLIOMYELITIS

At the present time, a diagnosis of poliomyelitis is made by the physician on clinical grounds, on chemical and cellular changes in the cerebrospinal fluid, on elimination of other forms of encephalitis, on the epidemiological background, and on the characteristic pathological lesions.

When we enter the field of laboratory diagnosis of this illness we are immediately confronted by barriers, some of which at this moment are insurmountable. In the first place, though a specific diagnosis can be made by the isolation and identification of the virus, such isolation is difficult. The virus can be recovered from the feces of the living patient who, in certain instances, harbors it for a few days before the acute attack, during the acute attack, and for weeks afterward. The recovery of virus from the pharynx of the patient during an acute attack is more difficult. Post-mortem, the virus can be recovered also from central nervous system. In view of its limited host specificity, expensive and rare monkeys are used in the isolation procedure, and in a number of instances the procedure may yield negative results, as will be shown. Dependence on recovery of the virus is not generally practical. Secondly, since most adults and many children may have undergone subclinical infection as may be revealed by the presence of serum antibodies, there is as yet no helpful serological test. Thirdly, there are different strains of poliomyelitis virus which are immunologically and serologically distinct. The important, basic factor of strains, which is indispensable for diagnosis, epidemiology, and knowledge of the entire poliomyelitis problem, has not as yet been completely, or even adequately, investigated. As it concerns our present subject, one may well inquire what particular strain shall be used for a neutralization test? There are other impediments in this field. For example, the serum neutralization test (no other serological test is available) is still carried out under prolonged incubation at 37°C. As will be shown in another paper, the question comes up whether this may not bring out cumulative, nonspecific inhibition rather than intensify or enhance specific neutralization.

It is proposed now to discuss some of the factors just mentioned which are involved in the laboratory diagnosis of poliomyelitis.

Isolation of virus: various strains. Failures to isolate virus from fatal human cases by transmission tests in animals, especially of the simian species, are numerous enough to attract attention. From 1909 to about 1930, when a great deal of such work was done in Europe and at the Rockefeller Institute, not more than 50 percent and 30 percent, respectively, of attempts were successful. In view of the fact that one of the outstanding properties of poliomyelitis virus is its limited host range, it was held that the virus in such negative cases may have been one that is transmissible only to man. If this were to be proved by more direct experimental methods, it should stimulate further effort to discover a means other than isolation of virus as a trustworthy laboratory aid to diagnosis (cf. Kessel *et al.* [18]).

In other instances, virus can be recovered from human beings by transmission tests in apes and lower monkeys, but not in other species of lower animals. The vast number of strains of virus now available in laboratories are of this category. These viruses show variable degrees of pathogenicity for monkeys—for example, the "dermal strains" of Trask and Paul, and the strains described by Flexner and Clark, and Kessel *et al.* (18) as possessing varying capabilities of infection by the intracerebral route. Strains have been reported as immunologically and serologically distinct from others, such as Philadelphia and M.V., Melbourne and M.V., Victoria and M.V., Rabaul and Massachusetts, Trask and Aycock, different Los Angeles strains, and others (18, 19). Systematic classification of the antigenic characters of the different strains, however, has not been attempted, although the need for such knowledge is great.

In still other instances, virus can be recovered from human beings which is transmissible not only to simian but also to rodent species, such as albino mice, cotton rats, and hamsters—the so-called Lansing strains, or rodent-adapted human poliomyelitis virus. While work is being actively pursued on successful transmission from human beings directly to rodents, their usefulness to replace monkeys for initial propagation of the virus is still undetermined. On record are the following types of Lansing virus: (a) Lansing, (b) MEF1, (c) SK or Y-SK of Doctor Paul's laboratory, (d) Ph., or Philips, of the same laboratory, (e) Koprowski-Norton-McDermott, the most recently isolated (20). Will the rodent-adapted strains offer an approach to the state in which mice can be used instead of monkeys for poliomyelitis research and thus open up the way for further investigations and possibly fruitful results? It appears that the Lansing type of virus is merely one of many distinct strains of poliomyelitis virus, reacting in its own way, producing its own homologous antibody. Recent studies by Brown and Francis (21) and by Hammon, Mack, and Reeves (22) have pointed to the fact that antibody to the Lansing strain did not represent an immune response to the virus responsible for the disease prevailing at the time. This view may find support in the recent work of Olitsky and Findlay (23), who reported that in Africa, where the MEF1 strain was recovered, all natives studied showed positive neutralization of MEF1 virus. While Brown and Francis (21) indicate that strains having the Lansing-type antigenic constitution do not, after a single infection, induce a persistent immunity to poliomyelitis but rather that repeated infection with them is common, Hammon et al. (22) state that it is far from being established that all of the antibody substances to the Lansing virus encountered in man or animals are due to contact with the poliomyelitis virus. Thus, more work is needed to determine, with respect to the antigenic complex, the relationship of one to another of the rodent-adapted strains, and, in addition, to find out the relationship of these antigenic constitutions to those of the monkey-adapted strains, and even to poliomyelitis itself.

Mention should be made of the fact that recent attempts in our laboratory to develop a complement-fixation test useful for diagnosis of infection with poliomyelitis virus have yielded results which are apparently hopeful, although no practical application can as yet be made. A certain, though incomplete, degree of fixation was noted: (a) in pooled sera (over 50 samples) of convalescent poliomyelitis, (b) in the serum of monkeys surviving infection with the MEF1 strain of poliomyelitis virus, and (c) in serum of mice immunized with mouse tissue containing active Lansing-type virus. The antigen comprised a concentrated extract of Lansing virus-infected mouse brain, from which the lipid fraction was removed. The protein moiety produced by precipitation with acetone-ether represented a concentration of about thirty-fold of this constituent over that present in untreated brain suspension. While this work was being pursued, a report by Loring, Raffel, and Anderson (24) appeared in which they showed that concentrated Lansing virus prepared by differential centrifugation specifically fixed complement in the presence of blood of rats immunized with formolized Lansing virus, and of the serum of monkeys and certain human beings convalescent from poliomyelitis infection.

Identification of the poliomyelitis virus. Even though the poliomyelitis viruses have not as yet been adequately identified and differentiated on the basis of antigenic constitution, they generally conform in other biological characteristics. Among these are the following:

a) Typical illness and poliomyelitic changes in affected man from whom the virus is recovered and in the disease induced in the experimental animal in which the virus has a high degree of neurotropism. Among rodent-adapted strains, disease is not produced in adult rodents by routes other than neural.

b) Marked animal species-specificity or limited host range.

c) Small size. They are among the smallest of all viruses.

d) High resistance to physical and chemical agents.

e) Low titer, or LD_{50}, as compared with other neurotropic viruses, that is, 10^{-3} or 10^{-4}, instead of 10^{-6} to 10^{-9}.

f) Noncultivability in series in developing chick embryos. Cultivation of some strains have been shown by Sabin and Olitsky (25) and by Burnet (26) to be successful only in human embryo tissue.

g) Serological and immunological reactions are characteristic. It is generally difficult to immunize by usual methods with these viruses as antigens, although the recent work of Morgan offers a method for classification of strains.

This list should be regarded as tentative; when more data become available, it is possible that additions to or subtractions from this list may be necessary.

Diseases of lower animals that resemble poliomyelitis in certain features. In the diagnosis of rodent-adapted strains of poliomyelitis, one must consider the fact that a spontaneous disease occurs in mice, the virus of which may be mistaken for a Lansing type. This disease was first designated by Theiler (27) as spontaneous encephalomyelitis of mice. Since there are other forms of murine encephalomyelitis, and since the pathological picture of the spontaneous disease is that of a poliomyelitis, this name, and also "murine encephalomyelitis" and "mouse, or murine, poliomyelitis" (poliomyelitis is commonly used to designate a human malady) are unsatisfactory. The virus of Theiler's disease, which was suggested as its proper name (28), is pathogenic for certain rodents only; it is immunologically distinct, in so far as can be ascertained by present methods, from poliomyelitis strains, but has properties in common with them.

A similar disease in swine is the Teschen, or Bohemian, disease, also called infectious swine paralysis and encephalomyelitis enzootica suum, or swine poliomyelitis. The virus of this infection has not as yet been studied completely. It is included here tentatively.

In connection with the diagnosis of rodent-adapted poliomyelitis virus one may encounter: (a) spontaneous diseases of the nervous system in rodents, other than Theiler's disease (29); (b) strains reported as isolated from poliomyelitis cases, which can be adapted to rodents and which do not conform with several of the general properties of poliomyelitis virus; and (c) viruses and diseases of a nature still unknown. Some of these agents correspond with the viruses of the encephalitis group (28, 29). More work is needed, especially on antigenic structure, to define more clearly the members of this group and the relationship of one to another and of each to poliomyelitis. An incomplete list of such strains is: SK and MM murine poliomyelitis (Jungeblut (30));[2] MV and Philadelphia, adapted to cotton rats (Toomey and Takacs (31)); the rat strains of Pearson et al. (32); Theiler's GDVII and FA viruses (27, 28, 29).

In this second part of the discussion, the neutralization and complement-fixation tests for the diagnosis of the encephalitis viruses will be described, particularly from the point of view of their limitations and the reservations that should be attached to interpretation of the results obtained.

NEUTRALIZATION TEST

In the neutralization test, serum and virus are mixed, kept as a rule at 37°C. for varying periods of time, usually two hours, and injected into susceptible animals. Several factors must be considered: serum-virus incubation, route of inoculation, species and type of animal, and appraisal of the results. These have already been described by the writers (5). No matter how the test is performed, the object is to achieve the greatest sensitivity and specificity.

Serum. Nonspecific components of this complex material may influence the results; no two sera, apart from their specific antibody content, can be said to be identical in all respects in the neutralization test.

Morgan, Whitman, and others have described a labile component which in varying degrees influences neutralization by enhancement of viral inhibition. This element can be removed by heat at 56°C., by prolonged storage at 2–4°C., or by dilution of the serum at not more than 1:5.

Another nonspecific effect may be produced by the action of the lipid component of serum. It has been shown recently (33) that lipids extracted from normal sera from several animal species can inactivate *in vitro* considerable amounts of virus, and furthermore, that the time

[2] After this lecture was delivered, J. Warren and J. E. Smadel (Fed. Proc., 1948, 7:311) reported that there is a serological relationship between the SK and MM strains and that of encephalomyocarditis virus, and as already stated in a prior section of this paper, there exists a serological relationship between the Mengo encephalomyelitis agent and the encephalomyocarditis, Columbia-SK and MM viruses. Thus it would appear as if a new group of encephalitis viruses, the members of which exist widely over the world, is being brought to light. Dick (personal communication) states that this group is not related to that comprising the poliomyelitis viruses.

needed for such inactivation is short, a few minutes being sufficient. Such inactivation occurs in the presence of serum and of serum proteins. Although the conditions under which this type of viral inactivation was effected did not duplicate exactly those of the neutralization test as usually performed, one cannot disregard the fact that serum lipid may be responsible for a certain degree of nonspecific action in the test. In a few neutralization tests in which lipid was added to some sera and extracted from other samples of the same sera, we observed differences in titer of between 0.2 and 0.8 log units; the difference was in general small, but one does not know whether it may add to that brought about by other nonspecific components. On the other hand, in tests with eight different human sera containing different amounts of lipid inactivation of virus could not be correlated with the amount of lipid in the sera.

Another factor which may influence the virus titer and thus simulate specific neutralization is pH of the serum, the effect of which is best noted when the serum is incubated at 37°C., and is increased with the length of time it is kept at this temperature. When a serum is incubated at 37°C. its pH increases to 8.5 or 8.7 in twenty-four hours. With the Japanese B virus it was found that the optimum pH for the virus at 37°C. in the presence of phosphate buffer was 7.0; pH values of 8.5 and 9.0 showed definite viral inhibition. Thus, a sample of the Japanese virus with a titer of 10^{-8} had the following titers after forty-eight hours at 37°C.; at pH 7.0, the titer was $10^{-6.5}$ and at pH 7.5 the titer was $10^{-4.5}$; at pH 8.0 and 8.5, no virus could be recovered at a dilution of 10^{-3}. A similar reduction in the titer of virus occurs when it is incubated with normal serum for similar periods. If, however, the serum has been buffered so that the pH remains at 7.0, there is no inactivation of virus beyond that which occurs, in the absence of serum, with phosphate buffer pH 7.0 alone. When, on the other hand, fresh serum, or fresh serum kept frozen, is used in a neutralization test, in which incubation of the serum-virus mixtures at 37°C. is carried out for two hours or less, the serum pH, usually about 7.3, does not change or influence the result.

Length of incubation period at 37°C. for the neutralization test. The results of recent studies in this laboratory would appear to show that in neutralization tests with Western and Eastern equine, West Nile, St. Louis, Japanese B and Russian Far East encephalitis, and the MEFI and Lansing poliomyelitis viruses, incubation for two hours at 37°C. as compared with nonincubation, produces a greater reduction in the titer of viruses. A similar degree of reduction occurs, however, whether specific antiserum or normal serum is added to the virus, and a somewhat lesser reduction with hormone broth. The degree of diminution of the titer of the viruses is not dependent on their original titers, whether low or high, or on the species of animal from which the serum is derived, or on the form in which serum is employed, such as stored in a refrigerator, or in the frozen state, or freshly prepared, or on the pH values of the serum or broth. Since the apparent increase in the neutralization index which is secured after preliminary incubation of serum-virus mixtures is not significantly greater than the amount of virus inactivated after incubation of normal serum-virus mixtures, and since this apparent increase in neutralization index may be nonspecific, the results would now indicate that incubation in the neutralization tests with the viruses mentioned is not necessary (34).

Virus. The way in which the virus is prepared and used in the neutralization test has already been described (5). Virus dilutions are mixed with undiluted serum or serum dilutions with a constant amount of virus. The method of serum dilution is superior if more exact determination of the degree of neutralization is desired. Its disadvantage is that the number of M.L.D. of virus used should be accurately calculated beforehand. It has been demonstrated by Horsfall (35) for influenza virus and by Morgan (36) for that of Western equine encephalitis that a linear relation exists between the dilution of serum and the dilution of the virus that is neutralized; the titer of serum will therefore vary with the amount of virus. For diagnostic use, the method of virus dilution with undiluted serum is more practical. Generally, 10 to 10,000 lethal doses of the encephalitis virus in tenfold dilutions are employed. This procedure should replace that in which only one dilution of virus is tested, as has been the practice in neutralization tests with poliomyelitis virus, especially with simian-adapted strains. Here, the procedure has been to inject few monkeys, sometimes only one, and to incubate undiluted-serum and virus mixtures at 37°C. overnight or for twenty-four hours—a technique that could yield problematical results. For research work, on the other hand, not only serum but also virus dilutions can be tested, in order to achieve more precise measurement of the neutralizing capacity of a serum, especially when it is desired to compare the capacity of one serum with that of another (35, 36).

Route of inoculation. A previous article (5) described the intracerebral and peripheral (intraperitoneal) routes of inoculation of susceptible animals, to test the degree of neutralization of virus by serum. The reservations for the intraperitoneal route, chiefly the need of unweaned mice, were stated, although it often is at least 10,000 times as sensitive an indicator of neutralizing capacity as the intracerebral route.

Reference should be made to the recent work (37) which describes the ratio between therapeutic and neutralizing doses of different types of infective agents, including neurotropic viruses. The therapeutic dose is determined by injecting serial dilutions of immune serum intravenously, and immediately afterward a constant amount of virus is introduced in skin, brain, or muscle. The neutralizing dose is measured by mixing serial dilutions of serum and a constant amount of virus *in vitro* and injecting 0.1 c.c. of the mixture into the same tissue. More work will be necessary before this ratio can be used as a means of diagnosis of the encephalitis and poliomyelitis viruses.

The precision of the appraisal of the degree of neutralization. When the result of a neutralization test is appraised, the first question is whether or not a given serum has significantly neutralized the virus (5). The problem is how to interpret neutralization or inhibition of small numbers of viral units, and whether such reactions are the result of sampling errors. It is generally stated, on arbitrary grounds, that neutralization indexes between 1 and 9 are negative; 10–49, equivocal; and 50 or more, positive. It is believed that a similar procedure to that used by Lauffer and Miller (38) for influenza and Horsfall and Curnen (39) for PVM might be of value for the viruses under discussion. The method consists in the determination for each virus, of the degree of reproducibility of infectivity titrations. If one is to know whether or not a difference of titer—for example, between $10^{-7.5}$ of an unknown serum and $10^{-8.5}$ of a control—is significant, it is first necessary to know how closely one can reproduce the $10^{-8.5}$ titer in the controls. All the intracerebral titrations with Japanese B encephalitis virus, twenty-five in number, done in our laboratory under comparable conditions during the past two years were analyzed by applying the statistical method reported (38, 39). A mean titer of $10^{-8.38}$ was found, with maximum deviations of $+0.82$ and -0.68. The variance was 0.149 and the standard deviation 0.387. Hence a difference in titer between any two suspensions equal to $2 \times \sqrt{2} \times 0.387 = 1.095$ log units shows that the probability that these two suspensions of virus are not identical is $p=.05$, ordinarily taken as significant. This value corresponds to a difference in neutralization index of 12 or 13. A greater difference would, of course, be still more significant. Were this analysis applied to simultaneous titrations of serial dilutions derived from the same original 10 percent suspension, the standard deviation would probably be smaller and the significance of small differences greater.

COMPLEMENT-FIXATION TEST

The complement-fixation test is the only *in vitro* test available for diagnosis of neurotropic virus infections. It is carried out by mixing antigen, serum, and complement, which are incubated together for a certain length of time; sheep red blood cells and antisheep hemolysin are then added; and after an additional short incubation at 37°C., the result of the test is recorded in terms of hemolysis or lack of it. It can be said, in general, that there is better agreement on the details of the complement-fixation test than on those of the neutralization test.

Antigen. Antigens are extracts of infected tissues, ordinarily mouse brain or chick embryo, treated to eliminate nonspecific and anticomplementary properties. As the different methods for preparing antigens have been repeatedly described (40), they will be only enumerated here: freezing and thawing, followed by centrifugation at 7,000 r.p.m.; centrifugation at 12,000 or 15,000 r.p.m.; extraction of lyophilized material with lipid solvents, preferably benzene, followed by moderate centrifugation; and, in the case of LCM, centrifugation at 30,000 r.p.m. By these methods the tissue components, particularly lipids, which are responsible for nonspecific reactions, are reduced or removed. Lipid-free antigens are apparently more satisfactory, and their availablity will facilitate the complement-fixation test. It is advisable to use avirulent antigens to prevent laboratory accidents; antigens can be inactivated by ultraviolet light, by heat, or by low concentrations of formalin.

Antigens prepared by the method of freezing and thawing had titers between 1:8 and 1:64 and were ordinarily used undiluted (40). For those prepared by newer methods, based on the technique of DeBoer and Cox, Espana and Hammon (41) report higher titers, even to 1:256 and 1:512. The question arises whether or not they should be diluted to save material. In our hands variation in amounts of antigen from 4 to 64 units made no appreciable difference in the titer given by a hyperimmune animal serum against the virus of Japanese B encephalitis. With antigens of higher titer, however, Espana and Hammon report that excess of antigen results in lower serum titers; they advise dilution of the antigen so that between 8 and 16 units are used. All antigens prepared by the methods mentioned above can be lyophilized and stored for long periods of time and still retain their properties unchanged. Whether these antigens are the virus particles themselves or soluble materials is of theoretical interest. The LCM antigen has been shown to be soluble; some observations on rabies led us to believe that that antigen too may be soluble.

Hyperimmune serum for control. Hyperimmune sera for standardization of antigens and for positive controls in the test are best prepared by immunizing animals with homologous tissue to minimize nonspecific and organ-specific reactions. This limits the preparation of sera to animal species which are susceptible to the virus. Moreover, the serum of animals which are apt to be anticomplementary or give nonspecific reactions—for example, rabbit serum—should not be used. The most satisfactory animals are mice, guinea pigs, and, perhaps, hamsters. Mice are susceptible to most of these viruses and thus have the advantage that uniformity can be maintained, which makes for better control; the amount of serum that is obtainable limits their use. Recently, Hammon and Espana (42) have reported that specific immune sera could be obtained from guinea pigs injected intracerebrally with mouse-propagated St. Louis and Japanese B encephalitis virus. Preparation of hyperimmune sera can best be achieved in mice or guinea pigs by repeated intraperitoneal injections—one or two doses of formolized virus, followed within a week or ten days by three or four injections of active virus in 10^{-2} dilution, given at intervals of a few days. By this schedule one can obtain high-titer sera in mice in three to four weeks; in guinea pigs, after a somewhat longer period.

Sera should be collected with a minimum of hemolysis; they can be kept indefinitely in the frozen state at $-76°C$.

Sera for test. Sera from patients should be collected aseptically, kept in lusteroid tubes or, better, in sealed glass ampules, and stored on dry ice until tested; this is, of course, the optimal procedure. The use of antiseptics, such as merthiolate (1:10,000) or phenyl mercuric borate (1:50,000), apparently does not interfere with the test.

Sera are first inactivated in order to destroy complement. Although the usual 56°C. for half an hour is sufficient in most instances, inactivation at 60°C. for twenty minutes is more satisfactory for human and mouse sera; the higher temperature does not appreciably affect the specific titer, and it removes minor anticomplementary and nonspecific reactions. For mouse serum the higher temperature is necessary, since it was found in many instances that the serum is anticomplementary even in a dilution of 1:8. Guinea-pig serum need not be inactivated at temperatures higher than 56°C. Wassermann-positive human sera react with brain-tissue antigens unless they are inactivated at 65°C. or unless the antigen is lipid-free. One can overcome this obstacle by other means, such as high-speed centrifugation of the antigen or filtration through Seitz pads, but these procedures are not so practical.

Complement. An accurate titration of complement in the presence of antigen is needed both preliminary to the test and along with the test. The titration during the test is performed so as to find the exact amount of complement present when the hemolytic system is added. With properly prepared antigens there is no anticomplementary effect; indeed, in some instances the degree of hemolysis may be slightly enhanced. The amount of complement in terms of units is of the first importance, since an excess will yield false negative results and a deficiency, false positive ones. Two units of complement is the optimal amount.

The hemolytic system. Sheep red blood cells and hemolysin are diluted to the desired strength and mixed half an hour before using. A sufficient amount should be prepared to permit the use of the same material for the preliminary titration of complement and for the test itself. While the first phase of the test at 4°C. for eighteen hours is going on, hemolysin and diluted sheep cells are kept in the refrigerator separately and mixed half an hour before being added to the tubes.

Other factors. There is evidence to indicate that in the first phase of the test, keeping the mixtures at 2–4°C. for eighteen hours is superior to short incubation—for example, one hour at 37°C. The titer of a serum given the longer incubation is often two to four times as high, and there are no anticomplementary or nonspecific effects. Each serum should be tested against several antigens similarly prepared, in order to ascertain the specificity of the test. Each serum should, of course, be tested also for anti-complementary reaction.

When it was necessary to conserve serum or reagents, the following volumes have been successfully used: 0.1 c.c. each of antigen, serum, hemolysin, and sheep cells, and 0.2 c.c. of complement containing two units, the total volume being 0.6 c.c.

The appraisal of each test must be based on the titer of complement in the presence of antigens and on the specificity of the reaction. It is important to realize that small, apparently insignificant anti-complementary or nonspecific reactions deriving from the different reagents may be cumulative and give false results. For this reason the use of numerous controls is always advisable.

REFERENCES

This is not a complete bibliography; a fuller list of references may be found in *A Bibliography of Infantile Paralysis 1789–1944*, ed. M. Fishbein (National Foundation for Infantile Paralysis, Inc., New York, 1946), and in the numerous excellent reviews of the subject recently printed, among them references 3, 9, 10, 12, 13, 16, and 19.

1. Rivers, T. M., and F. F. Schwentker, Louping ill in man, *J. Exp. Med.*, 1934, 59:669.
2. Casals, J., Immunological relationships among central nervous system viruses, *J. Exp. Med.*, 1944, 79:341.
3. Hammon, W. M., and W. C. Reeves, Recent advances in the epidemiology of the arthropod-borne virus encephalitides, *Am. J. Pub. Health*, 1945, 35:994.
    Reeves, W. C., Observations on the natural history of Western equine encephalomyelitis, *Proc. 49th Ann. Meet. U. S. Livestock Sanitary Commission*, Dec. 1945, pp. 150–158.
4. Olitsky, P. K., Epidemic, primary virus infections of the central nervous system of man, *Am. Nat.*, 1946, 80:401.
5. Olitsky, P. K., and J. Casals, Neutralization tests for diagnosis of human virus encephalitides, *J.A.M.A.*, 1947, 134:1224.
6. Sabin, A. B., R. W. Schlesinger, D. R. Ginder, and M. Matumoto, Japanese B encephalitis in American soldiers in Korea, *Am. J. Hyg.*, 1947, 46:356.

7. Burnet, F. M., D. Lush, and A. V. Jackson, The relationship of herpes and B viruses; immunological and epidemiological considerations, *Australian J. Exp. Biol. & Med. Sci.*, 1939, 17:41.
8. Sabin, A. B., Studies on the B virus, II: Properties of the virus and pathogenesis of the experimental disease in rabbits, *Brit. J. Exp. Path.*, 1934, 15:268.
9. Smadel, J. E., Research in virus diseases, *Bull. U. S. Army Med. Dept.*, 1947, 7:795.
10. Florman, A. L., Usefulness and limitations of laboratory studies in the diagnosis of virus diseases, *J. Mt. Sinai Hosp.*, 1947, 14:39.
11. Smadel, J. E., and M. J. Wall, A soluble antigen of lymphocytic choriomeningitis, *J. Exp. Med.*, 1940, 72:389.
12. Bedson, S. P., The laboratory diagnosis of virus infections of man; a review, *J. Clin. Path.*, 1947, 1:2.
13. Shwartzman, G., Some recent advances in bacteriology and virus research with special reference to electron microscopy, *J. Mt. Sinai Hosp.*, 1944, 11:137.
14. Beveridge, W. I. B., P. E. Lind, and S. G. Anderson, Mumps isolation and cultivation of the virus in the chick embryo, *Australian J. Exp. Biol. & Med. Sci.*, 1946, 24:15.
15. Enders, J. F., A summary of studies on immunity in mumps, *Trans. & Stud. Coll. Phys., Philadelphia*, 1945, 13:23.
16. Enders, J. F., Mumps; technique of laboratory diagnosis, tests for susceptibility and experiments on specific prophylaxis, *J. Pediat.*, 1946, 29:129.
17. Margulis, M. S., V. D. Soloviev, and A. K. Shubladze, Acute primary hemorrhagic meningo-encephalitis, *Am. Rev. Soviet Med.*, 1944, 1:409; An etiology and pathogenesis of acute sporadic disseminated encephalomyelitis and multiple sclerosis, *J. Neurol., Neurosurg., & Psychiat.*, 1946, 9:63.
18. Kessel, J. F., F. J. Moore, and C. F. Pait, Differences among strains of poliomyelitis virus in *Macaca mulatta*, *Am. J. Hyg.*, 1946, 43:82.
19. Aycock, W. L., Immunity to poliomyelitis; heterologous strains and discrepant neutralization tests, *Am. J. Med. Sci.*, 1942, 204:455.
20. Koprowski, H., T. W. Norton, and W. McDermott, Isolation of poliomyelitis virus from human serum by direct inoculation into a laboratory mouse, *Pub. Health Rep.*, 1947, 62:1467.
21. Brown, G. C., and T. Francis, Jr., The neutralization of the mouse-adapted Lansing strain of poliomyelitis virus by the serum of patients and contacts, *J. Immunol.*, 1947, 57:1.
22. Hammon, W. M., W. N. Mack, and W. C. Reeves, The significance of protection tests with the serum of man and other animals against the Lansing strain of poliomyelitis virus, *J. Bact.*, 1947, 57:285.
23. Olitsky, P. K., and G. M. Findlay, The use of rodent-adapted MEF1 strain of human poliomyelitis in neutralization tests with serum of apparently normal African natives, *J. Bact.*, 1946, 52:255.

24. Loring, H. S., S. Raffel, and J. C. Anderson, Complement-fixation in experimental and human poliomyelitis, *Proc. Soc. Exp. Biol. & Med.*, 1947, 66:385.
25. Sabin, A. B., and P. K. Olitsky, Cultivation of poliomyelitis virus *in vitro* in human embryonic nervous tissue, *Proc. Soc. Exp. Biol. & Med.*, 1936, 34:357.
26. Burnet, F. M., in *Directors Report, Walter and Eliza Hall Institute of Research in Path. and Med.*, Melbourne, Australia, 1938, 19:16.
27. Theiler, M., Spontaneous encephalomyelitis of mice, a new virus disease, *J. Exp. Med.*, 1937, 65:705.
28. Olitsky, P. K., Certain properties of Theiler's virus, especially in relation to its use as model for poliomyelitis, *Proc. Soc. Exp. Biol. & Med.*, 1945, 58:77.
29. For important data see Melnick, J. L., and J. T. Riordan, Latent mouse encephalomyelitis, *J. Immunol.*, 1947, 57:331.
30. Jungeblut, C. W., and M. Sanders, Studies of a murine strain of poliomyelitis virus in cotton rats and white mice, *J. Exp. Med.*, 1940, 72:407; Jungeblut, C. W., and G. Dalldorf, Epidemiological and experimental observations on the possible significance of rodents in a suburban epidemic of poliomyelitis, *Am. J. Pub. Health*, 1943, 33:169.
31. Toomey, J. A., and W. S. Takacs, Poliomyelitis virus acclimated to small laboratory animals, *Proc. Soc. Exp. Biol. & Med.*, 1941, 46:22.
32. Pearson, H. E., G. C. Brown, R. C. Rendtorff, G. M. Ridenour, and T. Francis, Jr., Studies of the distribution of poliomyelitis virus, III: In an urban area during an epidemic, *Am. J. Hyg.*, 1945, 41:188.
33. Casals, J., and P. K. Olitsky, Inactivation of certain neurotropic viruses *in vitro* by serum lipids, *Science*, 1947, 106:267.
34. Olitsky, P. K., and J. Casals, The effect of incubation at 37C on the neutralization test with various encephalitis viruses including Lansing strains of poliomyelitis virus, *J. Immunol.*, in press.
35. Horsfall, F. L., Jr., Neutralization of epidemic influenza virus; the linear relationship between the quantity of serum and the quantity of virus neutralized, *J. Exp. Med.*, 1939, 70:209.
36. Morgan, I. M., Quantitative study of the neutralization of Western equine encephalomyelitis virus by its antiserum and the effect of complement, *J. Immunol.*, 1945, 50:359.
37. Friedemann, U., Dynamics and mechanism of immunity reactions *in vivo*, *Bact. Rev.*, 1947, 11:275.
38. Lauffer, M. A., and G. L. Miller, The mouse infectivity titration of influenza virus, *J. Exp. Med.*, 1944, 79:197.
39. Horsfall, F. L., Jr., and E. C. Curnen, Studies on pneumonia virus of mice (PVM); the precision of measurements *in vivo* of the virus and antibodies against it, *J. Exp. Med.*, 1946, 83:25.
40. Casals, J., Complement-fixation test for diagnosis of human viral encephalitides, *J. Immunol.*, 1947, 56:337.

41. Espana, C., and W. M. Hammon, An improved benzene extracted complement fixing antigen for certain neurotropic viruses, *Proc. Soc. Exp. Biol. & Med.*, 1947, 66:101.
42. Hammon, W. M., and C. Espana, A simple method of producing control guinea pig immune sera for use with complement fixing antigens for the arthropod-borne virus encephalitides. *Proc. Soc. Exp. Biol. & Med.*, 1947, 66:113.

Chapter 7

THE DIAGNOSIS OF INFECTION WITH THE VIRUS OF HERPES SIMPLEX

By T. F. McNair Scott, Lewis L. Coriell, and Harvey Blank, *The Children's Hospital of Philadelphia, Department of Pediatrics and Department of Dermatology and Syphilology, School of Medicine, University of Pennsylvania*

The diagnosis of any virus infection depends in varying degree on the establishment of four criteria: (1) A characteristic clinical picture. (2) The isolation of the infecting virus. (3) A specific immunological response of the patient to that virus. (4) The presence in the patient's tissues of a pathological picture characteristic of that virus. In the diagnosis of herpetic infections it is often possible to establish all four criteria. However, in any given patient the diagnosis can be established on the basis of any combination of these, depending on the type of herpetic infection suffered.

The virus of herpes simplex has been quite extensively studied since it was first isolated from herpetic infections of the eye in 1912 by Grüter (1), and from the vesicles of herpes simplex in 1919 by Löwenstein (2). However, the present concept of the relationship of this virus to its natural host—man—has become clarified only within the last eight years through the pioneer studies of Dodd, Buddingh, and Johnston (3), and Burnet and Williams (4). Burnet (5) has pointed out that the herpes virus has evolved such an advantageous relationship with its human host that it is able to infect 90 percent of the population for 90 percent of their lives with little, if any, injury to them. True as this may be in the broad view of the biologist, as clinicians we have to take the narrower view of diagnosing those few instances in which the symbiotic relationship is not perfect, and manifest disease results.

The accompanying diagram indicates this present concept of the host-parasite relationship. An understanding of this is important because the criteria on which a diagnosis of herpetic infection is based will differ, depending on whether it is a primary or a recurrent in-

HOST-PARASITE RELATIONSHIP OF HERPES SIMPLEX VIRUS

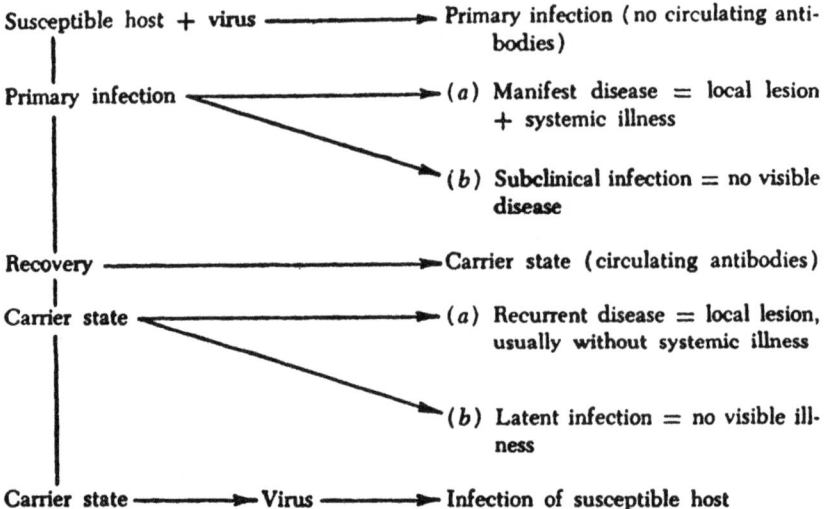

fection. In the former, characteristic local lesions, with a considerable systemic reaction, can often lead to a presumptive diagnosis, which can be established simply by demonstrating the development of circulating antibodies against the herpes virus on recovery. In the latter, a history of recurrence is common, and the local lesions are again often characteristic, usually without evidence of systemic reaction, so that a presumptive diagnosis can be made for this form also. However, only the isolation of virus or the demonstration of a characteristic histopathological picture can confirm the diagnosis. Immunological tests in this instance are useless because there is a high titer of antibodies during the clinical illness.

CLINICAL PICTURE

For the purpose of making a diagnosis, awareness of the variety of clinical conditions caused by this virus is important. A list of those at present recognized is given on page 85.

The primary infection is often subclinical, but when it is manifest it most frequently takes one of two forms: (a) an *acute herpetic gingivostomatitis* (6), which is a common clinical entity in any pediatric outpatient department, in children from one to three years, and which seldom causes difficulty in clinical diagnosis. This is only rarely

HERPES SIMPLEX

DISEASES CAUSED BY THE VIRUS OF HERPES SIMPLEX

Diseases of the Skin

Herpes simplex (various forms)
Eczema herpeticum (Kaposi)
Traumatic herpes

Diseases of the Mucocutaneous Junctions

Herpes labialis
Herpes progenitalis
Vulvovaginitis

Diseases of the Mucous Membranes

Acute gingivostomatitis
Recurrent stomatitis ?

Diseases of the Eye

Conjunctivitis
Keratoconjunctivitis

Diseases of the Central Nervous System

Meningo-encephalitis

a manifestation of recurrent herpes. (*b*) *Eczema herpeticum* (7), a rarer condition which occurs in persons, again usually children, with atopic eczema. In them, the injured skin becomes infected with the herpes virus. Differential diagnosis must be made from a similar lesion caused by vaccinia.

Primary herpetic vulvovaginitis (8) and *meningo-encephalitis* (9, 10) are less clinically specific, and diagnosis necessitates the demonstration of an immunological response to the herpes virus. Vulval herpes also occurs as a manifestation of the recurrent disease, but meningo-encephalitis has been reported only as a primary infection. There may be other clinical manifestations of primary infection not yet recognized. The problem of whether herpetic infection in the eye is ever primary is not yet clarified. Certain types of conjunctivitis, including membranous conjunctivitis associated with an enlarged, tender preauricular node, are recognized as herpetic, as are the more common forms of recurrent keratoconjunctivitis, of which dendritic ulceration of the cornea is the commonest of several types of corneal lesions (11). Virus can be isolated from such lesions and there are sometimes herpetic vesicles on the lids. The clinical features of some of these manifestations can be briefly reviewed.

The common *recurrent herpes* is characterized by a group of vesicles on an erythematous base, often at the mucocutaneous junctions of the lips.

Acute herpetic gingivostomatitis is a primary infection, often with history of exposure to an adult with a fever blister. The child has fever, painful lesions which are collapsed vesicles throughout the mucous membranes of the mouth, red swollen gums, submaxillary lymphadenopathy, and a fetid breath.

Eczema herpeticum (Kaposi's varicelliform eruption) is also usually a primary infection but may be recurrent. The eczematous areas of skin are covered with fresh and crusted vesicles, which on closer view can be resolved into typical grouped herpetic vesicles. These patients show marked and prolonged rises in temperature, as high as 105°F., and sometimes die of their disease. The recurrent disease manifests the same local lesions but causes much milder, if any, systemic illness, and runs a shorter course.

ISOLATION OF VIRUS

Herpes can quite readily be isolated from manifest examples of either primary or recurrent infections and also, at times, can be isolated from patients not suffering any apparent disease. Fluid from vesicles, swabs from mouth lesions, and saliva have frequently been shown to contain virus, and it has been isolated, at times, from brain, spinal fluid, and blood. There are three reliable methods for the isolation of the virus, which can be used in the laboratory: (*a*) inoculation of the chorioallantoic membrane of the embryonated hen's egg, (*b*) inoculation of the scarified cornea of the rabbit, (*c*) intracerebral inoculation of the rabbit and, probably less reliably, other animals, such as the mouse.

The first method has the advantage of being relatively inexpensive and, in our hands, has equaled in reliability the older and perhaps more commonly employed rabbit-cornea method. Any material can be used, but those from superficial lesions liable to be contaminated with bacteria must be made bacteriologically sterile. Saliva, or fluid specimens withdrawn into capillary tubes or a syringe through a fine needle, can be treated directly or diluted in a suitable diluent. In our hands, phosphate buffered saline pH 7.2, with ½ percent gelatine, is simple and effective. Nutrient broth and 10 percent rabbit serum saline can be used. Swabs from lesions are washed in the diluent. The saliva, fluid, or washings are allowed to stand in contact with one-tenth their volume of a solution containing 5,000 units of penicillin and 1,000 micrograms of streptomycin per ml., for one-half hour at room temperature. This sterilizes the majority of specimens. However, a small percentage of salivas are contaminated with the fungus of thrush,

Candida albicans. In this event, crystal violet 1:5,000 is added to the above antibiotic mixture. The final concentration of 500 units of penicillin, 100 micrograms of streptomycin, and 1:50,000 concentration crystal violet is harmless to the virus and to the egg membrane. After this preliminary treatment, the material is inoculated in 0.05 ml. amounts onto the chorioallantoic membrane of 10- to 13-day-old eggs. A false air sac is formed over the embryo, and the material is injected through a slit in the shell. Two eggs are inoculated and incubated at 96°F. for forty-eight to seventy-two hours. The membranes are then removed and examined against a dark background. If virus is present, characteristic plaques can be seen, either scattered or confluent, or the membrane is generally edematous. If no characteristic lesions are observed, passage is made through at least two more generations of eggs before being discarded as negative. Differential diagnosis from vaccinia is probably the most common difficulty. However, the plaques of herpes are small, very superficial, and often show an oval or a tailed form, in contrast to the larger, round, deeper plaques of vaccinia. In older lesions of both, central necrosis occurs, but again this is much more prominent in the vaccinial lesions. The histopathologic picture of the membrane at twenty-four hours is pathognomonic; it can easily be distinguished from that of vaccinia by the presence of the intranuclear inclusion bodies of herpes, which will be discussed later, and the more superficial involvement of the membrane in the herpetic lesion. In cases of doubt, a confirmatory neutralization test with known herpes and vaccinia immune sera must be performed.

The second method, using the rabbit's cornea, has been the standard since Grüter's first isolation in 1912. The advantage is that no preliminary treatment of the material is necessary to remove bacteria. It can be applied directly to the scarified surface of a rabbit's cornea. If virus is present, keratoconjunctivitis occurs within twenty-four hours to seven days after inoculation. This reaction is grossly indistinguishable from a positive Paul test caused by vaccinia virus. Exudate or the nictitating membrane contains virus and can be used for passage. The histopathologic picture of the cornea taken within twenty-four hours of the onset of symptoms is pathognomonic through the finding of the characteristic inclusion bodies of herpes and absence of those of vaccinia.

The third method is useful for such sterile materials as blood, cerebrospinal fluid, or brain emulsion. A volume of 0.25 ml. can be inoculated intracerebrally into a rabbit. If virus is present the rabbit will do one of three things: develop fever for several days, recover, and be immune to reinoculation with herpes virus; develop high fever for several days without other symptoms, and die suddenly; or develop signs of encephalitis, such as tremor, weakness of limbs, and drawing of the head to one side, and usually die. Histopathologic lesions with herpes inclusion bodies can be found in, and virus is recoverable from, the brains of such animals.

IMMUNOLOGICAL RESPONSE

This response can be determined by the neutralization test; or the skin test.

The neutralization test is the standard laboratory test for routine use. It can be done in two ways: in embryonated eggs and in mice.

The hen's egg technique provides an inexpensive, simple, and, with a little experience, reliable method of estimating the presence of herpetic antibodies. The technique as used in our laboratory is as follows, differing slightly from that described by Burnet (5): There is one point that should be made. In our hands it has not been found possible to preserve the egg-tissue virus well, so that a freshly passed virus not more than a week old is used as antigen. The virus is suitably diluted so that about 100 plaques are formed on the membrane. The paired, untreated sera to be tested are diluted 1:16 as is a control normal rabbit serum. The virus and sera are mixed in equal quantities and are incubated about an hour and a half in the icebox. The exact time does not appear to matter. Of each mixture 0.05 ml. is inoculated onto the chorioallantoic membranes of four eggs, which are then incubated at 96°F. for not more than forty hours. The development of satellite plaques after this time makes counting difficult. The membranes are removed and the plaques counted. The presence of antibodies is demonstrated by the reduction of the average plaque count of the four eggs of any serum mixture to less than 50 percent of the average count of the control. If a convalescent serum does not show the difference expected on clinical grounds, undiluted sera may be tested, which may then show a small antibody difference. This should be checked by testing further sera. However, the control serum should be kept at 1:16 dilution because undiluted normal rabbit serum at times depresses the plaque count nonspecifically—a phenomenon we have not encountered in undiluted normal human serum.

In the second method, the ordinary neutralization test, such as is used for the neurotropic viruses, is set up in mice. A 20 percent emulsion of infected mouse brain is incubated in decimal dilutions with equal amounts of undiluted sera to be tested. The 50 percent end point of each of the test sera is compared with that of the control serum and recorded in terms of the neutralization index. The mice usually have to be observed over a period of twenty-one days, and at least four mice have to be used for each serum-virus mixture. This makes the method more time-consuming and expensive than the previous method, but it is reliable and has become well standardized.

In the *skin test* the use of heat-treated herpes-infected amniotic or allantoic fluid as an antigen has distinct possibilities as a method of following antibody production. The few studies reported suggest that the presence of a positive skin test closely parallels the presence of circulating antibodies (12, 13). However, its use in actually following the development of antibodies in patients with primary herpetic infection has not been adequately studied. One of the difficulties in our hands has been the development of a stable antigen.

PATHOLOGICAL PICTURE

There are two characteristic, although not peculiar, pathological features of herpetic infection: (*a*) The presence of type A intranuclear inclusion bodies which can be found in any tissue, and (*b*) the ballooning type of degeneration which occurs in epithelial cells. Both these characteristics can be seen under high power in a section of a mucous membrane or skin lesion in which an inclusion body is often found in the nucleus of a greatly enlarged cell. The presence of these characteristics can be used as an aid to diagnosis of many types of skin or mucous membrane lesions suspected of being herpetic. With the "Keys cutaneous punch" a small portion of the lesion can be removed under local anesthesia with little discomfort to the patient. The specimen fixed in Bouin's solution can be embedded and stained with hematoxylin and eosin and will be ready for examination in three to four days. Under low power the characteristic skin vesicle shows its epidermal position and the presence of ballooning cells at the edge of the vesicle; in these, as stated, intranuclear inclusions can be found under higher magnification. The lesion of the mucous membrane shows the same features and, in its early stages at least, is really a collapsed vesicle and not an ulcer, as superficial clinical inspection might suggest. The pathological picture is indistinguishable from that of varicella and herpes zoster, and so is diagnostic only as confirmation of a characteristic clinical picture or in association with one of the tests discussed above.

SUMMARY

The establishment of a diagnosis of infection with the herpes simplex virus must depend first on clinical awareness of the varied clinical picture produced. In the primary infection the development of circulating and possibly tissue antibodies confirms the clinical impression; in recurrent infection confirmation must rest on the isolation of the virus or the histopathologic picture, or both.

REFERENCES

1. Grüter, W., Unpublished experiments, 1912: Experimentelle und Klinische Untersuchungen über den sogenannten Herpes corneae. *Ber. Versam. Deut. Ophth. Ges.*, 1920, 42:162.
2. Löwenstein, A., Aetiologische Untersuchungen über den fieberhaften Herpes, *Münch. med. Wschr.*, 1919, 66:769.
3. Dodd, K., J. Buddingh, and L. Johnston, Herpetic stomatitis, *J. Pediat.*, 1939, 25:105.
4. Burnet, F. M., and S. W. Williams, Herpes simplex. A new point of view, *Med. J. Australia*, 1939, 1:637.
5. Burnet, F. M., Virus as Organism (Harvard Univ. Monographs in *Med. & Pub. Health*, Cambridge, Mass., 1945).
6. Scott, T. F. M., A. J. Steigman, and J. H. Convey, Acute infectious stomatitis. Etiology, epidemiology, and clinical picture of a common disorder caused by the virus of herpes simplex, *J.A.M.A.*, 1941, 117:999.
7. Lynch, F. W., Kaposi's varicelliform eruption: Extensive herpes simplex as a complication of eczema, *Arch. Dermat. & Syph.*, 1945, 51:129.
8. Slavin, H. B., and E. Gavette, Primary herpetic vulvovaginitis, *Proc. Soc. Exp. Biol. & Med.*, 1946, 63:343.
9. Smith, M. G., E. H. Lennette, and H. R. Reames, Isolation of the virus of herpes simplex—demonstration of intranuclear inclusions in a case of acute encephalitis, *Am. J. Path.*, 1941, 17:55.
10. Armstrong, C., Herpes simplex virus recovered from the spinal fluid of a suspected case of lymphocytic choriomeningitis, *Pub. Health Rep.*, 1943, 58:16.

11. Gunderson, T., Herpes corneae with special reference to its treatment with strong solution of iodine, *Arch. Ophth.*, 1936, 15:225.
12. Nagler, F. P. O., A herpes skin test reagent from amniotic fluid, *Australian J. Exp. Biol. & Med. Sci.*, 1946, 24:103.
13. Rose, H. M., and E. Molloy, Cutaneous reactions with the virus of herpes simplex, *J. Immunol.*, 1947, 56:287.

Chapter 8

THE DIAGNOSIS OF RABIES

By HARALD N. JOHNSON, *The International Health Division, The Rockefeller Foundation*

History of exposure, clinical symptoms, and outcome of the illness often play an important part in the diagnosis of rabies. The disease in man commonly runs a rapid course with a fatal outcome within five days of the onset. Given a history of dog bite and the classical disease course with sensory symptoms referable to the site of exposure, intense excitation of the nervous system associated with convulsive seizures, and the hydrophobia symptom, terminating in death, it is evident that one is dealing with a case of rabies. Approximately 50 percent of the recognized cases of the disease occur among persons who have not been given the rabies vaccine treatment; in such cases the history of exposure ordinarily is obtained after the clinical symptoms have suggested the probability of infection with rabies. It is such a common thing for persons to be bitten by dogs that a minor wound so obtained may be forgotten or considered to be of no significance.

The acute phase of rabies follows one or another of the patterns exhibited by rabid animals; that is, some patients have a prolonged period of excitation, while in others depressive or paralytic symptoms are predominant from the beginning. In the former type the symptomatology may be similar to that of a variety of other diseases which cause encephalitis. The hydrophobia symptom is by no means a constant feature of this type of rabies. Difficulty in swallowing is a very common symptom, but until attempts to swallow precipitate painful spasmodic contractions of the muscles of the throat the patient will not exhibit fear of water. In cases of paralytic rabies it is especially difficult to make a clinical diagnosis, as the disease picture may be similar to poliomyelitis, paralysis following vaccine treatment, and other diseases which are associated with paralysis. Therefore, it is evident that not all cases of rabies are recognized as such. There is no proved instance of recovery from rabies in man; the disease is regarded as uniformly fatal. This appears to be true for cases exhibiting the classic disease course, but there is suggestive evidence that the paralytic type of rabies may not always be fatal. Koch (1) has described cases of what he believed to be abortive rabies, and there are many references in the literature to recovery from rabies. The failure to recognize recovered cases of rabies in man may be due to the fact that isolation of the virus in such cases depends on animal inoculation tests with saliva, which rarely are done even in suspected cases of rabies. Dogs inoculated intramuscularly with rabies street virus, in rare instances develop a paralytic disease and recover. There is no record of the isolation of rabies virus from the saliva in such cases, but infectivity studies have been limited to specimens taken after the acute phase of the disease has subsided. The vampire bat, *Desmodus rotundus murinus*-Wagner, is the only known vector of rabies that has been proved capable of acting as a carrier of the disease over an extended period without exhibiting evident illness, and recovery from rabies has been observed in this species (2). It is not unlikely that other species of animals may be able to transmit rabies as symptomless carriers in the same manner as vampire bats. There is some epidemiological evidence to suggest that the common rat, *Rattus norvegicus*, may be such a vector.

The laboratory diagnosis of rabies as now practiced is predicated on an expected 100 percent mortality rate for man and lower animals infected with the disease. The diagnosis is based on the finding at necropsy of Negri bodies in certain nerve cells of the brain or in the brains of laboratory animals inoculated intracerebrally with infected tissue from such cases. The development of diagnostic methods for determining whether animals are infected with rabies was necessitated by the frequency with which human beings are bitten by dogs. The principal emphasis is placed on observation of biting dogs for a period of at least seven days and examination of brain specimens from such animals should they die or be killed. This is done as an aid in advising whether or not vaccination should be recommended. In addition, it is necessary to examine specimens from all animals suspected of having the disease in order to limit the spread of rabies by quarantine or destruction of exposed dogs and cats and in order to have epidemiological information as to the extent of the disease. The reported incidence of rabies in animals, based on proved cases of the disease, is only an index of the extent of the infected area. The total number of animals dying of the disease is much higher. For example, in 1939 a study was made of the incidence of rabies among dead dogs picked up by sanitary department trucks in the city of Birmingham, Alabama (3). Over a period of seven months, 1,962 dead dogs were collected by the department of sanitation, and of these 477 were suitable for study. Rabies virus was isolated from 25 of these dogs, or 5.2 percent of those examined. During the same study period, 120 dogs suspected of having died of rabies were examined by the health department, and 50 were found positive for rabies. This study was carried on during a period of low incidence of rabies. The results would no doubt have been much more striking if the study could have been repeated in 1945 during a period of epizootic dog rabies. During the first five months of 1945 the sanitary department trucks picked up 8,528 dead dogs, and in May, which was the first month to show a sharp rise in the number of proved cases of rabies, they picked up 2,287 dead dogs. Only 34 proved cases of rabies were recorded in May of 1945.

Negri bodies cannot always be found in man and animals dying of rabies. Therefore, if the microscopic examination of a brain specimen is negative, it is necessary to resort to animal inoculation in order to establish the diagnosis. Diagnosis by this method is too time-consuming to influence the decision regarding vaccination of persons badly bitten. Animal inoculation serves principally as a confirmatory test in doubtful or controversial cases in which the clinical history of the offending or suspected animal is not consistent with the negative microscopic findings.

Negri bodies are readily demonstrated in impression preparations of brain tissue stained by the method of Sellers (4). Though Negri bodies usually are more abundant and characteristic in Ammon's horn than elsewhere in the brain, it is advisable to make preparations also from the cerebral and cerebellar cortices. The impression method is of particular value because the anatomical orientation of nerve cells is retained, and there is little distortion and rupture of cells. The Ammon's horn is exposed by cutting through the cortex over the posterior horn of the lateral ventricle. A section, 1 to 2 mm. in thickness, is removed from the middle of the horn, where it bulges up from the floor of the ventricle, and is placed on an absorbent surface.

such as a tongue depressor or paper toweling. Several impressions are obtained by touching a clean glass slide to the surface of the section. While still moist, the slide is immersed in the staining solution for about five seconds, after which it is washed in water. The preparation is ready for examination as soon as it is dry. Tap water, if not contaminated with certain mineral salts, is satisfactory for washing the stained preparation. If tap water cannot be used, uniform results are obtained by washing in M/150 phosphate buffer solution pH 7.0, prepared in distilled water.

Sellers' stain is made up as follows: Basic fuchsin, saturated absolute methyl alcohol solution, 2–4 ml.; methylene blue, saturated absolute methyl alcohol solution, 15 ml.; methyl alcohol, absolute, acetone free, 25 ml.

It is convenient to keep the staining solution in a Coplin jar which can be sealed with vaseline to prevent evaporation. Because of variability in the dye content of different lots of stain, an excess of the powdered dye should be used in preparing stock solution—for example, 4 gm. of basic fuchsin or 2 gm. of methylene blue to 100 ml. of absolute, acetone-free methyl alcohol. A properly stained smear, when light passes through it, should appear reddish-violet in thin areas and purplish-blue in thick portions. If, in the trial stain, the thin parts are bluish, add 0.5 ml. of the fuchsin solution. Negri bodies are stained cherry red and stand out in sharp relief; the basophilic inner structure is colored deep blue. The cytoplasm of nerve cells is stained blue to purplish-blue; nuclei and nucleoli are deep blue; the stroma is rose-pink, and nerve fibers are colored a deeper pink; neural sheaths are not stained; bacteria, if present, are stained deep blue; and erythrocytes are copper color. For the demonstration of Negri bodies in paraffin sections, brain tissue should be fixed in Zenker's fluid containing 5 percent glacial acetic acid, and the sections should be stained with phloxine-methylene blue or Wolbach's modification of Giemsa's stain as described by Mallory (5).

In human specimens there is little chance of making a mistake by confusing the inclusion bodies of rabies with those which occur in other diseases. In dog brains, however, inclusion bodies caused by distemper virus may be encountered which are similar to those occurring in rabies. The distemper inclusion bodies are pale red, are more refractile than those caused by rabies, and have no inner structure.

They may be irregular in outline, and occur more frequently in the thalamus and lentiform nuclei than in Ammon's horn. Intracytoplasmic inclusion bodies may be found in the brains of mice which do not have rabies. These are small, pink to bright red in color, very refractile, and uniformly round; they have no inner structure.

The diagnosis of rabies by isolation of the virus depends on injection into animals of saliva taken during the disease or brain tissue obtained at necropsy. An attempt should be made to isolate the virus from saliva of human beings suspected of having rabies, particularly those suffering from the paralytic type which is difficult to differentiate from the paralysis caused by rabies vaccine. Since the submaxillary salivary glands are most likely to contain virus, specimens of saliva should be taken from under the tongue. Undiluted saliva is apt to cause immediate death when injected intracerebrally into laboratory animals, but it may be given intramuscularly. For this type of test inoculation, the guinea pig is the animal of choice. For intracerebral test inoculation in mice, the saliva should be diluted 10^{-1} and 10^{-2} in saline containing at least 2 percent inactivated normal guinea pig serum and penicillin in a concentration of at least 1,000 units per ml.; both dilutions should be tested.

Brain tissue obtained at necropsy should be preserved in undiluted neutral glycerol; portions of the medulla, basal ganglia, and cerebral cortex should be used. If the disease was of long duration, there may be little or no virus in the brain. There is considerable variation in the distribution and concentration of virus in various sections of the cerebral cortex, spinal cord, and nerve trunks of human beings dying of rabies. The spinal fluid rarely contains virus (6). Fresh or glycerolated specimens of brain tissue are prepared for inoculation by grinding in a mortar and adding normal saline solution to make a 10 percent suspension. The supernatant fluid following centrifugation is used for inoculation of mice. When bacteria are seen in preparations, small portions of the brain should be placed in glycerol for a few days, or, if it is necessary to avoid delay, the tissue may be suspended in normal saline solution containing 0.5 percent phenol and stored at 4°C. for twenty-four hours before testing. The virus may be separated from bacteria by filtration. It will pass through diatomaceous earth and unglazed porcelain filters which withhold common varieties of bacteria, but much of it is retained in such filters unless the tissue-virus suspension is subjected to a preliminary clarification by passing it through a coarse filter. Penicillin may be used for counteracting bacterial contamination.

Methods for the isolation and identification of rabies virus have been known for a long time. Until a few years ago the guinea pig and the rabbit were considered the most suitable animals for infectivity studies. Recent studies have shown that the white laboratory mouse is the best experimental animal for the isolation of rabies virus (7, 8). The advantages of the mouse are its low cost, making possible the use of several animals for the testing of one specimen; the relatively short incubation period of rabies in this animal; and the consistency of the production of Negri bodies in the brains of mice inoculated intracerebrally with street rabies virus. Any of the various strains of white mice are equally suitable as test animals (9). There is no significant decrease in susceptibility to intracerebral infection with increasing age. If the specimen is positive, some of the mice ordinarily will show tremors, incoordination, or paralysis from six to eight days after inoculation. Convulsive seizures are a common symptom, and the animal may die during such a seizure. Most mice infected with the natural virus develop flaccid paralysis of the legs, which progresses to complete prostration. Frequently, Negri bodies can be demonstrated in the brain five days after inoculation. The incubation period may be prolonged to two or three weeks; this is most apt to occur when the virus is present in low titer, as is apt to be the case if the disease was of long duration. It is necessary to confirm a diagnosis of rabies in mice by finding Negri bodies, since several viruses, as well as some bacterial and protozoal diseases, produce a disease picture in this species similar to that of rabies.

Rabbits and guinea pigs may be used for diagnostic inoculation. In general, the incubation period of rabies caused by street virus is fifteen to thirty days for rabbits and ten to twenty days for guinea pigs when the virus is introduced into the brain. At times, the incubation period may be as long as ninety days. The disease in rabbits and guinea pigs is similar to that described in mice.

Negri bodies can be found in approximately 70 percent of human cases of rabies (10). The duration of symptoms before death has a definite correlation with absence or abundance of Negri bodies. This substantiates the widely accepted procedure of holding a suspected

TABLE 1

SUMMARY OF MICROSCOPIC AND MOUSE-INOCULATION STUDIES OF DOG BRAINS, GEORGIA STATE DEPARTMENT OF HEALTH, 1937

Month	Negri +	Negri 0	Mouse + Negri 0	Total +	Percentage of Total Positive That Was Negri 0
January	62	37	5	67	7.5
February	50	38	1	51	2.0
March	67	48	13	80	16.2
April	76	48	6	82	7.3
May	77	93	7	84	8.3
June	58	76	9	67	13.4
July	73	68	8	81	9.9
August	39	63	11	50	22.0
September	48	39	4	52	7.7
October	45	35	6	51	11.8
November	53	45	7	60	11.7
December	42	33	4	46	8.7
Total	690	623	81	771	10.5

animal until death rather than killing the suspect. Table 1 shows the results of microscopic and mouse-inoculation studies of dog-brain specimens received by the Georgia State Department of Health during 1937. Of 1,313 brain specimens tested, rabies virus was isolated from 771, of which 690 were positive for Negri bodies (10). This indicates that a positive microscopic diagnosis can be made in approximately 90 percent of biting dogs infected with rabies.

Suggestive evidence of variation in the strains of virus was obtained; this was based on the ability of the different strains to promote the formation of Negri bodies when tested in dogs. Some strains nearly always produced a paralytic disease in experimentally infected dogs, and the infection was characterized by a rapid course and absence of Negri bodies. In this connection it may be noted that 26 percent of the thirty-five brains of rabid foxes, which were obtained during the peak month of an epizootic, contained no Negri bodies, while all the brains of fifty-nine foxes obtained during the subsequent enzootic phase of the outbreak, were shown to contain both virus and Negri bodies (10, 11).

Animals examined for rabies are usually those which develop the excited type of the disease, and become vicious and bite. Dogs developing the paralytic type of rabies are not apt to be examined, as ordinarily there is no question of human exposure. Among dogs infected experimentally with street virus, some die suddenly without showing signs of excitation, and, as a rule, about 50 percent of them develop the paralytic type of the disease and seldom live more than one or two days after the onset of the illness. Less than 50 percent of such infections are characterized by the formation of Negri bodies (10). It is during the early stages of the disease that animals are particularly dangerous, as they may appear alert, friendly, and even unusually affectionate but will bite at the slightest provocation. It is likewise the wild animal that loses its timidity of man that must be suspected of rabies.

When characteristic Negri bodies cannot be demonstrated in the brains of mice infected with a virus otherwise characteristic of rabies virus, it may be identified by determining whether or not it is neutralized by rabies-immune serum (7, 8). The complement-fixation test is applicable to the study and identification of rabies virus (12).

Serological methods for the diagnosis of rabies are available; that is, both the neutralization and complement-fixation tests are applicable to the diagnosis of this disease. It should be a standard practice to take blood serum samples at the first opportunity in cases of suspected rabies, as well as in all types of encephalitis. A rise in titer of specific antibodies may be demonstrated during the disease course despite a fatal termination. There is also the possibility of recovery from rabies, and unless serological methods of diagnosis are applied, there is little chance of obtaining a definite diagnosis in the absence of clinical signs suggestive of rabies infection. Therefore, serological methods for the diagnosis of rabies should be included among the tests carried out on acute and convalescent phase serum specimens in all otherwise unidentified cases of encephalitis or encephalomyelitis. It is true that the rabies vaccine treatment does stimulate the production of specific serum antibodies, indistinguishable from those produced by natural infection. However, it has been mentioned previously that only about 50 percent of the recognized cases of rabies occur among persons given the vaccine treatment. Isolation of the virus from the saliva is the only method of identifying a nonfatal case of paralytic rabies from one of paralysis occurring as a result of the vaccine treatment. Recovery of rabies virus from the saliva by animal inoculation is a practicable method of diagnosis, and a recent case report illustrates the importance of this method of diagnosis (13). The virus is not present in the saliva of all cases of rabies. The demonstration of Negri bodies in the brain or isolation of the virus from this organ depends on a fatal termination and permission for post-mortem examination. The application of serological methods of diagnosis may prove to be useful in identifying cases of rabies where other means fail or cannot be done, as well as furnishing the first evidence that it is possible for man to experience infection with rabies and recover.

REFERENCES

1. Koch, J., "Lyssa," W. Kolle, R. Kraus, and P. Uhlenhuth, *Handbuch der pathogenen Mikroorganismen* (Berlin, 1930), VIII, 547–673.
2. Pawan, J. L., Rabies in the vampire bat of Trinidad, with special reference to the clinical course and the latency of infection, *Ann. Trop. Med.*, 1936, 30:401.
3. Denison, G. A., and C. N. Leach, Incidence of rabies in dogs and rats as determined by survey, *Am. J. Pub. Health*, 1940, 30:267.
4. Sellers, T. F., A new method for staining Negri bodies of rabies, *Am. J. Pub. Health*, 1927, 17:1080.
5. Mallory, F. B., *Pathological Technique*, pp. 86, 195 (Philadelphia, 1938).
6. Leach, C. N., and H. N. Johnson, Human rabies, with special reference to virus distribution and titer, *Am. J. Trop. Med.*, 1940, 20:335.
7. Webster, L. T., and J. R. Dawson, Early diagnosis of rabies by mouse inoculation, measurement of humoral immunity to rabies by mouse protection test, *Proc. Soc. Exp. Biol. & Med.*, 1935, 32:570.
8. Webster, L. T., Diagnostic and immunological tests of rabies in mice, *Am. J. Pub. Health*, 1936, 26:1207.
9. Johnson, H. N., and C. N. Leach, Comparative susceptibility of different strains of mice to rabies virus, *Am. J. Hyg.*, 1940, 32:38.
10. Johnson, H. N., The significance of the Negri body in the diagnosis and epidemiology of rabies, *Ill. Med. J.*, 1942, 81:383.
11. Johnson, H. N., Fox rabies, *J. Med. Assn. Ala.*, 1945, 14:268.
12. Casals, J., and R. Palacios, The complement fixation test in the diagnosis of virus infections of the central nervous system, *J. Exp. Med.*, 1941, 74:409.
13. Duffy, C. E., P. V. Woolley, Jr., and W. S. Nolting, Rabies; a case report with notes on the isolation of the virus from saliva, *J. Pediat.*, 1947, 31:440.

Chapter 9

THE DIAGNOSIS OF DENGUE[1]

By R. Walter Schlesinger, *Division of Infectious Diseases, The Public Health Research Institute of The City of New York, Inc.*

WHILE RECENT SUCCESS in the propagation of dengue virus in laboratory animals gives promise that this disease may eventually be readily diagnosed by simple laboratory procedures, progress thus far made does not permit an outline of specific diagnostic measures for general use. The clinical and epidemiological aspects of the disease are usually sufficiently well defined to allow differentiation from other febrile illnesses. Nevertheless, more specific tests may reveal that what is called typical dengue in some areas is actually a different disease. Also, the occasional occurrence of dengue in "atypical" forms has undoubtedly at times caused diagnostic difficulties.

CLINICAL FEATURES

Dengue is characterized by a striking discrepancy between the prostrating subjective symptoms and the negligible mortality rate. Fever usually lasts five to seven days. Anorexia, severe headache, intense aching and pains "all over," with special predilection for the lower back, extremities, and retro-orbital space, are practically always present. In addition, there may be a multitude of other symptoms referable to various organ systems, such as: change in the sense of taste, nausea, vomiting, constipation, severe abdominal distress, coryza, sore throat, and rarely, mental changes, especially depressive states, during convalescence.

In experimental transmission studies on dengue, where fully susceptible human beings are infected by the natural mode, that is, the bite of infected *Aedes aegypti,* one is struck by the observation that a more or less pronounced generalized rash is practically always recognizable. The rash is usually morbilliform, sometimes scarlatini-

---

[1] Most of the information contained in this discussion is based on recent studies by Sabin and by Sabin and Schlesinger. Details of these studies await publication. Two reports by these authors that have been published are listed at the end of this paper.

form, in character and is in some instances superseded by localized petechial eruptions. It usually arises during the latter half of the febrile period.

Lymph nodes are enlarged but not tender. During the first two to three days of fever, there is a marked increase in the number of immature neutrophile leukocytes ("shift to the left") with a normal or slightly reduced total white-cell count. Later, the total count goes down, often to around 2,000, and there may be relative lymphocytosis.

EPIDEMIOLOGICAL CONSIDERATIONS AND THE PROBLEM OF IMMUNITY

Many of these clinical features are shared by other febrile diseases. Dengue must be suspected if such cases appear in the presence of one of the transmitting mosquito species, A. *aegypti*, A. *albopictus*, and possibly A. *scutellaris*. There is no evidence to suggest that dengue has ever occurred in the absence of one of these vectors. However, even in known or suspected endemic areas, "dengue-like" fevers of as yet unknown etiology have made their appearance from which it has not been possible to isolate a virus by inoculation of acute-phase blood into human subjects.

On the other hand, in bona fide outbreaks of dengue, cases have been seen in which the course was unusually short and mild, and rashes were absent. Sabin has been able to show that similar mild cases can be produced experimentally in partially immune persons. The occurrence of repeated attacks, whether typical or not, had led many authors to the assumption that dengue did not result in immunity. However, even earlier epidemiological studies, such as those of Siler and associates (1) in the Philippines in 1922, suggested very strongly indeed that the native population in an endemic area does derive a considerable degree of protection from past and probably repeated exposures to dengue virus. These authors compared the incidence of dengue in native Philippine soldiers with that among recently arrived American soldiers. At the height of the epidemic season, there were about 450 cases per 1,000 of the latter, while the incidence among the natives remained negligible throughout the year.

Sabin's recent studies have brought out more clearly that recovery from an attack of dengue can, indeed, lead to complete and prolonged immunity. The picture is, however, complicated by the existence of multiple immunological strains of the virus.

DENGUE

By inoculation into human volunteers of acute-phase blood obtained from patients in the field, Sabin isolated seven strains of dengue virus. Of these, one originated in Hawaii, four in New Guinea, and two in Calcutta, India. Active immunity tests revealed that the Hawaiian, the two Calcutta, and one of the New Guinea strains were immunologically indistinguishable. Recovery from an attack caused by any one of these strains led to solid and lasting immunity to the others. However, the other three strains isolated from cases occurring on New Guinea, designated as New Guinea B, C, and D, while related to the Hawaiian-type virus, were not identical with it. When Hawaiian dengue-convalescent individuals were reexposed within several months to one of these New Guinea strains, or vice versa, second attacks of the disease ensued in most cases; but some of them were quite mild, lasting only one to three days, and characterized by the absence of rash. It has become clear from these studies—and this has been confirmed by serological tests in mice which will be discussed below—that at least two heterologous types of dengue virus exist. It is of special interest that heterologous strains were isolated from cases occurring during the same season in New Guinea.

EXPERIMENTAL TRANSMISSION OF DENGUE TO MAN

In all these experiments of Sabin on human volunteers, the identification of isolated strains of virus was based on the production of the typical disease and on its transmission from man to man by the bite of *A. aegypti*. The disease can also be produced by intracutaneous, subcutaneous, intramuscular, or intravenous inoculation of blood obtained from a patient during the acute phase, preferably during the first twenty-four hours of fever, when 1 ml. of blood has been found to contain as many as 1 million minimal infective doses of virus. Intracutaneous inoculation of the virus is followed after three to five days by the development of a local erythematous lesion, but this simple test is unsuitable as a routine diagnostic procedure because it invariably produces the disease.

THE USE OF THE MOUSE IN THE DIAGNOSIS OF DENGUE

Prospects for the development of more feasible and routinely applicable laboratory tests for the diagnosis of dengue have brightened since it was found possible to propagate dengue virus in the brains of laboratory mice and to carry out neutralization tests in these animals. However, it is well to preface the discussion of this phase by pointing to certain difficulties which have thus far impeded progress: (a) The adaptation of any strain of human dengue virus to the mouse is a tedious procedure, and repeated attempts were unsuccessful even with those strains which finally were established in the new host; (b) despite repeated efforts, it has not yet been possible to propagate all available strains in mice.

Various breeds of mice differ in their susceptibility to dengue virus. The best results in primary transmission attempts with human virus have been obtained in two- to three-week-old "dba" mice from Bar Harbor. On the other hand, a strain of albino mice bred through many generations at the Rockefeller Institute in Princeton was found much less susceptible to mouse-adapted virus than "Swiss albinos" obtained from a dealer. When this latter strain was used for the adaptation of the Hawaiian strain of dengue virus, at most one or two of ten mice inoculated intracerebrally with human dengue serum showed suggestive signs of disease after varying incubation periods. The incidence of manifest disease did not consistently rise above that rate for seven to eight consecutive mouse-to-mouse passages in which 10 or 20 percent suspensions of brain and spinal cord from weak or paralyzed mice served as the inocula. Only after fifteen such passages did the incidence of paralysis rise to 100 percent, and the virus finally reached infective titers of the order of 10^{-4} after several additional passages. With increasing numbers of passages, the mortality also rose to practically 100 percent, and the incubation period in mice, initially variable but mostly about three weeks in duration, became stabilized around nine to fourteen days, depending on the concentration of virus injected.

When the virus had finally attained this degree of adaptation to the mouse, the disease in this species differed little from those caused by a number of other neurotropic viruses, such as 17D yellow fever, and Theiler's mouse encephalomyelitis. It differed, particularly from the latter, by its limited host range: cotton rats, hamsters, rabbits, and guinea pigs could not be infected. Its identification as dengue virus was initially based on the production of a markedly modified form of dengue in man following the inoculation of the mouse-adapted

DENGUE

virus, which resulted in solid immunity to unmodified human dengue virus of the homologous type.

As the Hawaiian virus attained higher degrees of infectivity for the mouse, it became possible to utilize it for neutralization tests. Sera of monkeys inoculated with either human or mouse-adapted Hawaiian virus neutralized the latter. Specific antibody was also produced in rabbits. In human serum, after experimental infection, type-specific neutralizing antibody was found to be demonstrable on the first day after defervescence and for at least two years thereafter. Sera obtained from persons who had the spontaneous disease in Hawaii two years previously, similarly neutralized the mouse-adapted virus. Sera taken after longer intervals have not as yet been tested.

The technique of the neutralization test, as performed thus far, has followed the pattern used with certain other viruses. Stock virus was prepared in the form of 20 percent crude suspensions of infected mouse brain and spinal cord in whole or 50 percent inactivated (56°C. for thirty minutes) rabbit serum. It retained its titer for several months when stored in the dry-ice chest. An adequate number of ampoules containing the stock suspension were stored in this manner so that a fresh ampoule could be used for each neutralization test. All sera to be tested were likewise stored in the dry-ice box. Serial tenfold dilutions of virus were mixed with equal parts of undiluted test serum, and the mixtures were incubated for two hours in the 37°C. water bath. The mixtures were then inoculated intracerebrally into groups of five to ten mice. The results obtained were expressed in terms of the "neutralization index" for each serum, that is, the antilog of the difference between the titers of virus in the presence of normal and of the test serum.

To date, the other strains of dengue virus have not been sufficiently well adapted to the mouse, or their immunological pattern has not been sufficiently clarified, to permit their use in the development of routine diagnostic tests.

Neutralization of the mouse-adapted Hawaiian virus by homologous antibody manifests itself in two ways: (a) 50 to 1,000-fold reduction in the titer of the virus, (b) significant prolongation in the incubation period of those mice which do become paralyzed. Effects in the same direction have been noted in tests with sera from individuals convalescent after experimental infection with one of the heterologous strains (New Guinea B, C, D); but these results have been sufficiently variable in magnitude to limit the present practical usefulness of the test to the diagnosis of cases caused by the Hawaiian type of virus. In this manner, the test has been put to limited use in epidemiological surveys. For the serological diagnosis of individual cases, as for similar tests in other virus diseases, it is essential that at least two suitable serum specimens be available, one taken during the acute phase or as shortly thereafter as possible, the other later in convalescence. Demonstration of neutralizing antibody in the latter will be indicative of recent infection only if it is not demonstrable, or is present on a lower level, in the first specimen.

To assure the proper evaluation of results obtained with acute-phase serum, it is important to mention an "interfering" effect upon the mouse-adapted virus which has been observed in tests with serum taken from experimental cases of Hawaiian dengue within twenty-four hours after onset. Such sera, as will be remembered, contain large amounts of unmodified virus. In mixtures of such sera with suitable dilutions of mouse-adapted virus, the titer of the latter may be reduced to a degree compatible with type-specific neutralization. However, in those mice which become paralyzed the incubation period is not prolonged. In an attempt to differentiate this effect of acute-phase serum from the neutralizing action of convalescent serum, both were heated at 56°C. for thirty minutes. Unfortunately, this resulted in apparent loss of neutralizing antibody as well as of the interfering factor of acute-phase serum. However, while effective neutralization of the virus by specific antibody requires incubation of the serum-virus mixtures for two hours at 37°C., the interfering effect of acute-phase serum was equally strong with or without such incubation. It is probable that the unmodified human virus present in high concentration in such sera is responsible for this interfering action, comparable to similar phenomena described for other virus combinations.

CONCLUSIONS

The foregoing discussion has been limited to a review of the present knowledge of the etiological agent of dengue. It is clear that more convenient and surer methods of isolating and adapting the virus from human cases and further delineation of naturally occurring antigenic types are required, before any procedure can be readily applied to clinical and epidemiological surveys. At this early stage, it seems probable that such methods will be forthcoming.

Since dengue is a nonfatal disease for which there is no known treatment, it is doubtful whether laboratory methods for its diagnosis in individual cases will be much in demand. The principal importance of such tests will clearly be confined to the field of public health in connection with epidemic outbreaks and in endemic areas, and to the wider problem of differentiating true dengue from other diseases characterized by similar syndromes.

REFERENCES

1. Siler, J. F., M. W. Hall, and A. P. Hitchens, Transmission of dengue fever by mosquito, *Philippine J. Sci.*, 1926, 29:1.
2. Sabin, A. B., and R. W. Schlesinger, Production of immunity to dengue with virus modified by propagation in mice, *Science*, 1945, 101:640.
3. Sabin, A. B., Dengue (p. 289) in *Diagnostic Procedures for Virus and Rickettsial Diseases*, American Public Health Association (New York, 1948).

Chapter 10

THE DIAGNOSIS OF INFECTIOUS MONONUCLEOSIS

By JOHN R. PAUL, *Section of Preventive Medicine,
Yale University School of Medicine*

THE ETIOLOGICAL AGENT of infectious mononucleosis is as yet undiscovered, but it has become customary to regard this hypothetical agent as a virus. The disease will probably remain in the category of virus diseases until proved otherwise.

Clinically the diagnosis is reached via at least three channels: (*a*) the clinical examination of the patient; (*b*) the cytological examination of the blood; and (*c*) the serological determination of the titer of antibodies in the patient's serum against sheep erythrocytes. No one of these methods should be used to the exclusion of the others, and all of them should be evaluated in relation to the chronological stage of the disease. Thus, although infectious mononucleosis is characterized by general glandular enlargement, by mononucleosis, and by an increased titer of sheep cell agglutinins, yet none of these signs may be present in the first week of the disease, whereas one, two, or all three may appear more or less simultaneously during the early part of the second week.

We shall not be concerned in this report with the first method of diagnosis, namely, an evaluation of clinical signs, but only with the blood counts and the serological tests.

BLOOD COUNT

There are wide variations in the total white-cell count in infectious mononucleosis, but there is a general pattern which can be related to various stages of the disease. Irregularities in this pattern result from the fact that it is often difficult to determine accurately the day of onset of the disease. Furthermore, the duration of illness is variable, ranging from a few days to three weeks or more.

Leukopenia, which is a granulocytopenia, is common early. In a series of eighty-six cases personally reviewed (1) the total white-cell count was below normal in about 40 percent of the counts made between the fourth and tenth days of the disease, ranging from 5,000 per cu. mm. to as low as 2,000 per cu. mm. Leukopenia is apt to be followed in the second week by a moderate leukocytosis averaging from 10,000 to 15,000; the highest count (noted on the twentieth day of the disease) in our series, was 44,000 white blood cells.

The granulocytes remain more or less reduced in numbers for at least two weeks, the leukocytosis just mentioned (prominent between the tenth and the seventeenth day) being due largely to an increase in lymphoid cells. (See Table 1.) This increase in lymphoid cells seems to gather momentum about the eighth or ninth day. Owing to the variable character of the disease it is not possible to say how long the leukocytosis lasts—perhaps two weeks on an average.

TABLE 1

DIFFERENTIAL LYMPHOID CELL COUNTS IN 86 PATIENTS SEEN IN THE NEW HAVEN HOSPITAL (1938–45) AND LISTED ACCORDING TO THE DAY OF THE DISEASE

First Week		Second Week		Third Week	
Day of Disease	Percentage of Lym. Cells	Day of Disease	Percentage of Lym. Cells	Day of Disease	Percentage of Lym. Cells
1	46.4	8	41.5	15	69.9
2	31.3	9	50.1	16	54.2
3	32.9	10	55.9	17	60.7
4	37.1	11	71.0	18	52.5
5	42.2	12	55.5	19	46.4
6	45.2	13	57.5	..	..
7	40.1	14	53.0	21	53.0
Average	39.1		55.2		57.2

The predominating mononuclear cell which has been designated as characteristic of infectious mononucleosis is a lymphocyte; a varying number of these cells are distinctly abnormal. They are usually large, often showing foamy or deeply basophilic cytoplasm, many with fenestrations or vacuoles[1] (2). Although there may be difficulty in

[1] The mere presence of lymphoid cells of this type, which may occur in the absence of other signs, is not diagnostic of infectious mononucleosis. Randolph and Hettig (3) have stressed this point in their studies. They have reported the fairly frequent finding of atypical lymphocytes characteristic of those observed in infectious mononucleosis, in the peripheral blood of individuals who had a variety of allergic conditions.

classifying these cells when stained by Wright's method, the supravitally stained preparations show the majority to be large lymphocytes. The usual blood stains, such as Wright's stain, are adequate, however, for the average study of blood films in these cases.

In general, therefore, the blood picture of this disease is an exaggeration of a response familiar in a variety of acute febrile diseases of virus origin. Influenza, measles, mumps, sand-fly fever, dengue fever, and in particular infectious hepatitis—all show in varying degree granulocytopenia in the earlier stages of illness, followed by a moderate increase in lymphocytes, either with or without a leukocytosis. The picture differs in infectious mononucleosis only in that after the granulocytopenia, the outpouring of lymphoid cells into the blood stream is more pronounced than in the other acute febrile diseases mentioned, and many more atypical lymphocytes are included among the increased mononuclear cells.

SEROLOGICAL PROCEDURES

The sheep cell or heterophile agglutination test for the diagnosis of infectious mononucleosis is a *nonspecific* type of serological reaction perhaps in the same class as the Wassermann reaction in the diagnosis of syphilis, or the Weil-Felix reaction in some of the rickettsial infections. Its origin rests on the following historical data: In 1917 Friedemann (4) demonstrated the presence of sheep erythrocyte antibodies (presumably Forrsman's heterophile antibody) in normal human sera. Taniguchi (5) and others, notably Davidsohn (6), found that antibodies (presumably Forrsman's in type) for sheep erythrocytes were considerably increased in serum sickness. Paul and Bunnell (7) showed that an appreciable increase in sheep cell agglutinins occurred in infectious mononucleosis. Bunnell (8) later pointed out that this finding was sufficiently consistent to allow the test to be used for the diagnosis of this disease. It was assumed at first that the heterophile antibody of infectious mononucleosis was of the Forrsman type, but Bailey and Raffel (9) and Stuart (10) subsequently found that the sheep cell agglutinins in infectious mononucleosis could be differentiated from those of serum sickness and from those of normal serum. Sheep cell agglutinins in infectious mononucleosis are completely absorbed by beef erythrocytes, but are not reduced significantly by absorption with guinea pig kidney. Sheep cell agglutinins in serum sickness are completely absorbed by both guinea pig kidney and beef erythrocytes. Sheep cell agglutinins in normal human serum are not ordinarily absorbed by beef cells but are completely or almost completely absorbed by guinea pig kidney (see Table 2). The antigenic fractions of beef cells and guinea pig kidney which absorb their respective antibodies are thermostable, so that boiled or even autoclaved cells and tissue can be used for differential absorption tests. An explanation for the presence of this particular type of heterophile antibody in infectious mononucleosis is still obscure.

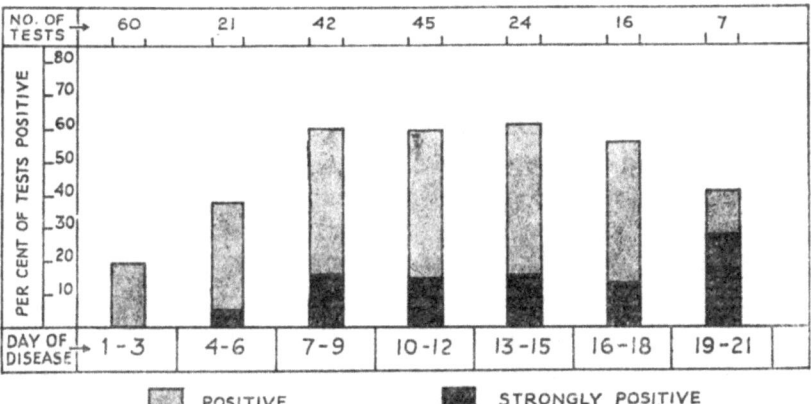

FIGURE 1. THE RATIO OF POSITIVE AND STRONGLY POSITIVE HETEROPHILE ANTIBODY TESTS IN A SERIES OF 81 PATIENTS SEEN AT THE NEW HAVEN HOSPITAL
From Gardner and Paul (1)

Two methods will be outlined: (a) the standard technique as outlined by Stuart (11) and modified slightly by the Connecticut State Health Laboratories; and (b) a qualitative, micro method recently described by Evans (12).

Standard method. It is desirable to have matched specimens of serum, the first taken as soon as infectious mononucleosis is suspected, the second taken in the second week of the disease, and the third taken during the third or fourth week after the onset of the disease. (See Fig. 1.) If only one specimen is available it may yield more valuable information if obtained in the second or third week of the disease than if obtained in the first week.

Blood is drawn as for a Wassermann test (5 to 10 ml. is desirable).

serum is separated from the clot by centrifugation, removed, and inactivated at 56° for thirty minutes. Inactivation is indicated because some normal sera possess a relatively high lytic titer for sheep cells.

For the antigen a 1 percent suspension of sheep erythrocytes, washed with physiological saline at least three times, is used. Freshly washed cells are desirable. Citrated blood (10 vols. of blood in 12 vols. of sterile 3.8 percent sod. citrate sol.) may be kept for a week. For serial tests blood from the same sheep should be used when possible.

Twofold serial dilutions (1:2.5 to 1:1280) of inactivated serum in amounts of 0.5 ml. each with an equal volume of 1 percent sheep red blood cell suspension yields a final serum dilution of 1:5 to 1:2560, and all titers should be reported on this basis. For a control, 0.5 ml. of the cell suspension is added to 0.5 ml. of saline. The tubes are incubated at 37°C. in the water bath for two hours and then placed in the icebox overnight. Readings are made the following morning after shaking, and the highest final serum dilution showing visable agglutination is taken as the titer. It is essential that the tests be read after the times specified.

There is some disagreement in the literature concerning the diagnostic titer of sheep cell agglutinins in infectious mononucleosis serum, and this can be explained, in part at least, by the fact that variable techniques have been used. Titers which range from 1:10 to 1:40 should be considered negative; titers from 1:80 to 1:160 are suspicious; and agglutination titers of 1:160 or more are considered as definitely elevated and may be referred to as positive. The best criterion in the early stages is that of a rising titer.

For the absorption test to differentiate types of heterophile agglutinins, Stuart's method (11) is advocated.

Absorbing agents. By the use of guinea pig kidney tissue and beef erythrocytes, three types of sheep cell heterophile agglutinins can be identified in human serum. Usually absorption with guinea pig kidney is sufficient for a final diagnosis of infectious mononucleosis, but, particularly when there is a question of lymphatic leukemia, a subsequent absorption with beef cells proves the agglutinins to be of the infectious mononucleosis type.

Fresh guinea pig kidney or portion of kidney is finely minced and ground in a hand or mechanical mortar, and the emulsion is strained or rubbed through a small piece of 13 xxx bolting cloth or its equivalent. Ten to 15 ml. of distilled water are added to the emulsion in a centrifuge tube. This is spun at 3,000 r.p.m. for about fifteen minutes and the supernatant particles, especially fat particles, discarded. This washing operation is repeated three or four times. The sediment is diluted with saline to a turbidity of at least twice that of barium sulfate turbidity standard No. 10.

Dried guinea pig kidney may be more convenient. It is prepared by grinding the kidneys in a fine meat chopper and washing in distilled water as described above. The washed macerate is dried in an evaporating dish at approximately 75°C., with frequent stirring to prevent caking. The tissue emulsion can also be dried by lyophilization. The dried macerate is finely ground in a ball mill or by hand in a mortar, then sifted through 13 xxx bolting cloth, and stored in a dry place.

In using dried tissue an amount of the powder sufficient to give a turbidity of at least twice that of the barium sulfate turbidity standard No. 10 is added to 1 ml. of saline and thoroughly wetted. This takes several minutes and should not be hastened.

Beef cells. Serum is removed from defibrinated beef blood by washing three or four times with saline. The packed cells are used for the absorption test.

Absorption tests. One ml. of guinea pig kidney suspension is added to 1 ml. of a 1:2.5 dilution of the serum to be tested. The mixture is incubated at 37°C. for thirty minutes in either a water bath or an air incubator and centrifuged at 4,000 r.p.m. for fifteen to twenty minutes. The supernatant fluid is then tested in serial dilutions for sheep cell agglutinins, as previously described. It is essential that the supernatant fluid be clear after centrifugation, since strong turbidity may inhibit agglutination of the sheep cells (10). If agglutinins remain, further confirmation of infectious mononucleosis can be obtained by a second absorption with beef cells. To 1 ml. of the serum dilution adsorbed with guinea pig kidney 0.5 ml. of packed beef cells is added, mixed, and incubated at 37°C. in either a water bath or an air incubator for thirty minutes. After centrifugation the supernatant fluid is tested for sheep cell agglutinins as before.

The relationships of the different types of sheep cell agglutinins in human serum are shown in Table 2. Agglutinins, which may be present in normal serum to a titer of 1:160, and in serum sickness, to a

Table 2

AGGLUTININS FOR SHEEP ERYTHROCYTES IN HUMAN SERUM

Type of Serum	Unabsorbed	Agglutination of Sheep Erythrocytes	
		Absorbed with Guinea Pig Kidney	Absorbed with Beef r.b.c.
Normal	− or +	−	Unchanged
Infectious mononucleosis	+	+	−
Serum sickness	+	−	−

titer of 1:20,480, are removed by absorption with guinea pig kidney. Absorption with beef cells alone is not advised, since this will not distinguish between infectious mononucleosis and serum sickness, and, as Davidsohn (6) has shown, sheep cell agglutinins may persist in the blood for a year or more after treatment with horse serum. The failure of guinea pig kidney to affect the sheep cell agglutinin titer of the patient's serum is adequate evidence of infectious mononucleosis; and so, removal by beef erythrocytes of the agglutinins remaining after absorption with guinea pig kidney is a final confirmation seldom required.

Qualitative rapid micro method. Evans (12) has recently described a rapid micro method for heterophile antibody determination using capillary blood and a white-cell pipette. This rough but valuable test may serve as a *screening* method. The patient's whole blood is used instead of serum, and the heat inactivation step is omitted. Absorption tests are not included. The method is as follows:

Capillary blood is drawn from the patient up to the 0.5 mark in a standard white-cell pipette and diluted to the 11 mark with normal saline.

This mixture is placed in a small test tube, measuring approximately 7 cm. in length and 0.7 cm. in diameter, and an equal volume of saline is added by refilling the white-cell pipette to the 11 mark.

The tube is centrifuged at approximately 2,000 r.p.m. for one to two minutes.

The supernatant fluid is drawn up to the 11 mark on the white-cell pipette and then mixed with an equal volume of 1 percent sheep red blood cell suspension in another small tube.

The test tube is centrifuged as before at 2,000 r.p.m. for one to two minutes and then shaken or struck sharply with the tips of the fingers until the sediments themselves become dislodged from the bottom of the tube. If definite evidence of agglutination is seen after thorough shaking, the test is recorded as "positive"; if no agglutination is visible, and the red blood cells become resuspended, the test is recorded as "negative."

The use of the terms positive and negative appears justified since the equivalent titer in this simplified test roughly corresponds with a serum dilution of 1:160, which has been taken as diagnostic in the standard method. It should be mentioned that a dilution equivalent to 1:80 can be obtained merely by drawing blood up to the 1 mark on the white-cell pipette and proceeding as described.

While only the designations positive and negative are used in reporting results from this test, a rough estimate of the actual titer in terms of serum dilution can be gained by observation of the type of agglutination. High-titer serum results in a tightly packed mass of agglutinated red blood cells that is dislodged easily from the bottom of the tube but tends to remain in large clumps on shaking. Titers in the low "positive" range of 1 to 1:160 and 1:320 result in more finely dispersed agglutinated particles; and titers in the high normal range 1:80 suggest agglutination when the tube is first agitated but rapidly go into suspension.

It is important to indicate that the heterophile antibody test is not always positive in infectious mononucleosis, and, in fact, figures on this point differ widely in different series. In our own series of eighty-one patients the test was positive in the first week of the disease in from 20 to 40 percent of the cases. In the second week of the disease the test was positive in about 60 percent of the cases and in the fourth week, in considerably less than 60 percent. (See Fig. 1.) The important feature is that a fair percentage of the cases can be diagnosed on grounds other than that of a positive heterophile antibody.

SUMMARY

The common laboratory tests for the diagnosis of infectious mononucleosis include (a) the examination of the total number and character of the patient's white blood cells; and (b) the determination of the titer of sheep erythrocyte agglutinins in the patient's serum, which should be accompanied by certain absorption tests. The agglutination methods proposed by Stuart (11) are described as a standard test, including the technique for absorption tests with guinea pig kidney and beef erythrocytes. A qualitative micro method proposed by Evans (12) is also described, which is of some value as a screening test.

REFERENCES

1. Gardner, H. T., and J. R. Paul, Infectious mononucleosis at the New Haven Hospital, 1921–1946, *Yale J. Biol. & Med.*, 1947, 19:839.
2. Osgood, E. E., Fenestration of nuclei of lymphocytes; a new diagnostic sign in infectious mononucleosis, *Proc. Soc. Exp. Biol. & Med.*, 1935. 33:218.
3. Randolph, T. G., and R. A. Hettig, The coincidence of allergic disease, unexplained fatigue, and lymphadenopathy; possible diagnostic confusion with infectious mononucleosis, *Am. J. Med. Sci.*, 1945, 209:306.
4. Friedemann, U., Über heterophile Normalamboceptoren; ein Beitrag zur Lehre von der Entstehung der normalen Antikörper, *Biochem. Ztsch.*, 1917, 80:333.
5. Taniguchi, T., Studies on heterophile antigen and antibody, *J. Path. & Bact.*, 1922, 25:77.
6. Davidsohn, I., Heterophile antibodies in serum sickness, *J. Immunol.*, 1929, 16:259.
7. Paul, J. R., and W. W. Bunnell, The presence of heterophile antibodies in infectious mononucleosis, *Am. J. Med. Sci.*, 1932, 183:90.
8. Bunnell, W. W., A diagnostic test for infectious mononucleosis, *Am. J. Med. Sci.*, 1933, 186:346.
9. Bailey, G. H., and S. Raffel, Hemolytic antibodies for sheep and ox erythrocytes in infectious mononucleosis, *J. Clin. Invest.*, 1935, 14:228.
10. Stuart, C. A., Heterophile antibodies in infectious mononucleosis, *Proc. Soc. Exp. Biol. & Med.*, 1935, 32:861.
11. Stuart, C. A., Infections mononucleosis, in *Diagnostic Procedures and Reagents; Technics for the Laboratory Diagnosis and Control of the Communicable Diseases* (2d ed., New York, 1945).
12. Evans, A. S., A simplified "qualitative" method for heterophile antibody determination using capillary blood and a white cell pipette, *J. Lab. & Clin. Med.*, 1947, 32:1278.

Chapter 11

THE DIAGNOSIS OF EPIDEMIC, MURINE, AND SCRUB TYPHUS, AS WELL AS Q FEVER

By Joseph E. Smadel, *Department of Virus and Rickettsial Diseases, Army Medical Department Research and Graduate School, Army Medical Center*

THE UNDERLYING PRINCIPLES employed in the laboratory diagnosis of epidemic and murine typhus, scrub typhus, and Q fever are similar to those used for this purpose in other infectious diseases. The first method, from a historical point of view, is isolation of the agent. Blood specimens drawn from patients during the early febrile phase of the illness, or tissues obtained at autopsy, contain the agents of all four diseases; the isolation of these rickettsiae is accomplished by inoculating guinea pigs or mice with such materials.

The response elicited in guinea pigs inoculated with blood from typhus cases is graphically illustrated in Fig. 1. *Rickettsia burneti*, the causal organism of Q fever, and *R. tsutsugamushi*, the agent of scrub typhus, also induce febrile diseases in guinea pigs; these are not accompanied by scrotal swelling. The animal generally chosen for recovery of the rickettsiae of scrub typhus is the mouse rather than the guinea pig. The identification of a rickettsial agent, once it has been recovered, is a lengthy and involved process. I shall not discuss these aspects because isolation and identification of these agents are no longer required as diagnostic procedures except perhaps in scrub typhus. Furthermore, the handling of animals and materials infected with these agents is hazardous to laboratory personnel; indeed, the isolation of *R. burneti* should not be attempted except by immune workers actively engaged in the study of this problem.

The Weil-Felix reaction is a useful, simple procedure which can be performed accurately in any hospital laboratory. The demonstration of the development of agglutinins against the OX-19 and OX-2 strains of *Bacillus proteus* justifies a presumptive diagnosis of infection with the agent of epidemic or murine typhus, or of spotted fever. The Weil-Felix reaction does not enable one to differentiate between epidemic and murine typhus, and it offers only suggestive data for differentiating between the typhus fevers and spotted fever. The reaction is of value in scrub typhus, in which agglutinins appear for the OX-K

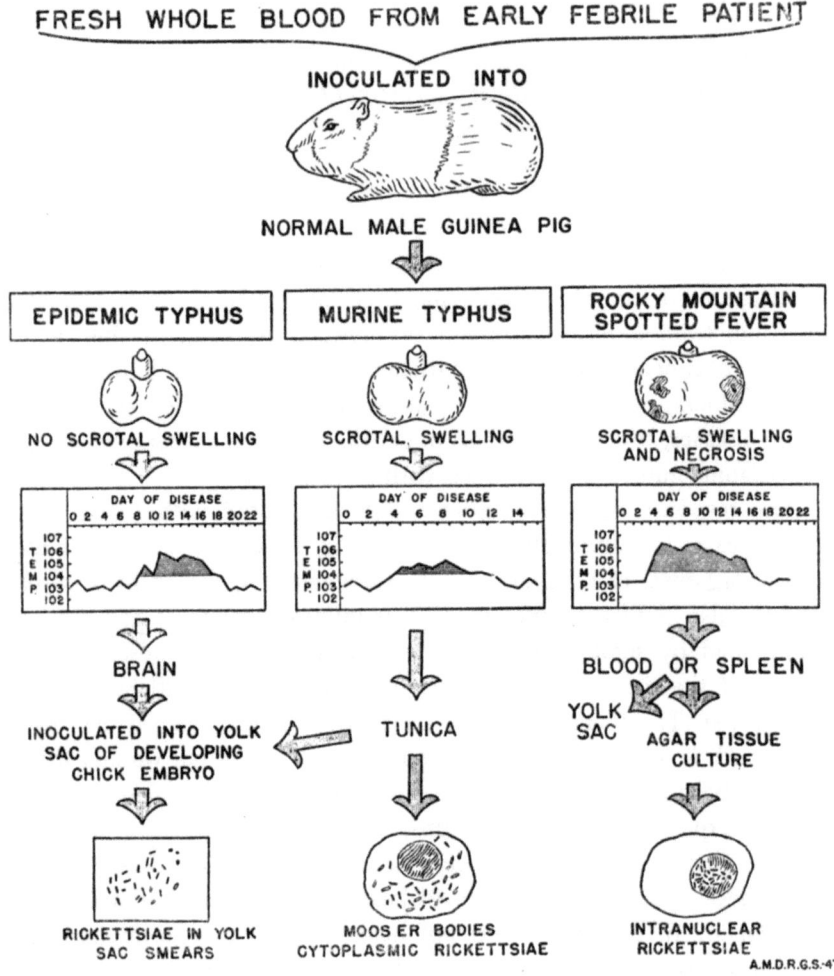

FIGURE 1. ISOLATION OF RICKETTSIAE
From *Diagnostic Procedures for Virus and Rickettsial Diseases*, American Public Health Association (New York, 1948)

strain but not for the OX-19 and OX-2 strains. In Q fever no agglutinins develop against any of the three proteus organisms. The usual results obtained with the Weil-Felix reaction in these diseases are

TABLE 1
USUAL WEIL-FELIX AGGLUTINATION REACTIONS OBSERVED IN RICKETTSIAL DISEASES[a]

Disease	OX-19	OX-2	OX-K
Epidemic typhus	++++	+	0
Murine typhus	++++	+	0
Scrub typhus	0	0	++++
"Q" fever	0	0	0
Rocky Mountain spotted fever	++++	+	0

[a] Reproduced from Plotz (1).

summarized in Table 1 (1). The test performed in tubes with serial dilutions of serum and constant amounts of proteus suspensions is recommended; the results are expressed as the highest dilution of serum which aggregates the test organisms.

It may be mentioned that other methods of determining proteus agglutinins are extremely useful to field workers and to investigators interested in typhus. These include the rapid slide method of Castañeda (2), which employs a drop of finger blood; the rapid test-tube reaction of León (3), and other modifications of the standard procedure. Still other special methods employ the demonstration of a specific antigen of typhus which appears in the urine (León [4]) or the blood (Smorodintseff and Fradkina [5]) of patients early in the disease, before the appearance of the rash and before the development of specific antibodies.

Patients with epidemic or murine typhus develop agglutinins for the proteus OX-19 organism between the fifth and the eighth day. The titer of antibody rapidly rises, generally reaching a peak during the third week, and drops off rather quickly. This early appearance of antibody, combined with the simplicity of the test, accounts for the continued employment of the Weil-Felix reaction in the diagnosis of typhus. It is extremely important, in using this serological test, that several samples of serum be examined at different periods of the illness, since it is of greater diagnostic import to show a rise in titer of OX agglutinins than it is to demonstrate the mere presence of such agglutinins. Actually, a positive Weil-Felix reaction obtained on a single sample of serum is of little value unless the titer is high, that is, above 1:320. The Weil-Felix reaction, like the Wassermann reaction, the Paul-Bunnell test, and others, is nonspecific in the sense that the antigen used to detect antibodies in the patient's blood is not the etiological agent.

During the past few years specific serological methods for the diagnosis of epidemic and murine typhus and Q fever have been widely employed. These methods consist of complement-fixation or agglutination techniques in which purified rickettsial antigens are used in tests with the patient's serum. A number of procedures have been used for preparing the antigens and testing the sera. These methods have been reviewed in detail elsewhere (6) and need not be discussed except to summarize briefly the general principles. Antigens consisting of partially purified suspension of R. prowazeki, R. mooseri, and R. burneti are prepared from infected yolk sacs of embryonated eggs in the following manner: The crude infected yolk sac tissue suspension is inactivated with formaldehyde and freed of considerable amounts of yolk fat by ether extraction, and then the rickettsiae are washed by differential centrifugation. This washing procedure is important in the preparation of specific typhus antigens. Plotz and his co-workers (7) have pointed out that certain closely related rickettsiae, such as the agents of epidemic and murine typhus and the agents of spotted fever and boutonneuse fever, contain common soluble antigens. If these are not removed by washing or by some other method, then the resultant antigens cannot be used to differentiate between these closely related infections.

The typical serological response of patients with epidemic typhus fever is illustrated in Fig. 2 (7). These graphs represent the average titers obtained by rickettsial complement-fixation and agglutination tests, with sera taken on alternate days from a group of thirty-two cases of epidemic typhus studied in Cairo in 1943 and 1944 by members of the U.S.A. Typhus Commission and the Army Medical School (7). Complement-fixing antibodies which react with the rickettsiae of epidemic typhus begin to appear in small amounts during the second week after onset of fever and rapidly increase, reaching a maximum titer at about the end of the third week. In contrast, when the same type of rickettsial antigen is used in agglutination tests, antibodies are detectable at an earlier date, that is, toward the end of the first week; these also reach their peak titer during the third week. It may be noted in the rickettsial agglutination graph that data are given for the tests made with both epidemic and murine rickettsial antigens. In these cases the titers were always sufficiently higher with epidemic antigen to prevent difficulty in interpreting the type of infection which occurred. A few of the sera, when tested with murine antigen by the complement-fixation technique, also gave positive results, but this occurred only with very low dilutions of serum. In Fig. 2 the anti-

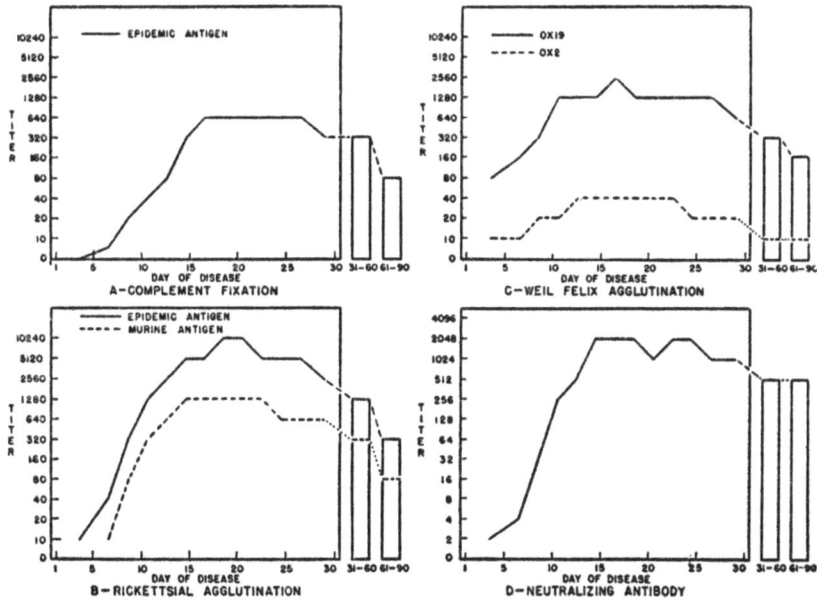

FIGURE 2. SEROLOGICAL RESPONSE OF 32 CASES OF EPIDEMIC TYPHUS FEVER BY DAY OF DISEASE, EXPRESSED AS RECIPROCAL OF MEANS OF TITERS
From Plotz et al. (7)

body response of the typhus patients as determined by two other techniques is presented graphically. Immune substances capable of neutralizing the toxin of epidemic typhus appear about the same time as do the rickettsial agglutinins. I shall not discuss the neutralization test because it is of little value in the diagnosis of this disease; the technique is too laborious and expensive. The development of agglutinins against OX-19 and OX-2 strains of B. proteus is also presented graphically in Fig. 2. These antibodies appear and reach a peak at about the same time as do the specific rickettsial agglutinins.

The serological response of a group of cases of murine typhus studied in Nashville, Tennessee, by members of the Army Medical School is presented in Fig. 3 (8). The general pattern here resembles that observed in epidemic typhus. The complement-fixing antibodies which react with washed murine rickettsiae appear toward the end of the second week and increase until about the end of the third. Very few of the patients developed antibodies detectable in the complement-

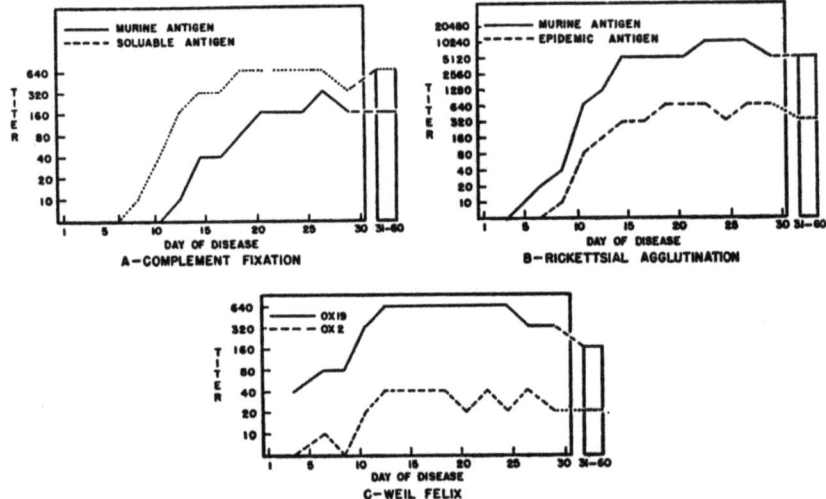

FIGURE 3. SEROLOGICAL RESPONSE IN 15 CASES OF MURINE TYPHUS FEVER, GEOMETRICAL MEAN OF TITERS BY DAY OF DISEASE
From Scoville et al. (8)

fixation test employing epidemic rickettsial antigen, and in the few instances in which such antibodies appeared, they were in low dilutions. The response as determined in rickettsial agglutination tests resembles that in epidemic typhus in that the sera are capable of agglutinating both murine and epidemic rickettsiae. However, the titers are always higher in the test employing R. mooseri. The toxic substances associated with the agents of murine typhus and epidemic typhus are closely related immunologically but are not identical. The pattern of development of neutralizing antibodies capable of inactivating the toxic effect of R. mooseri is essentially the same in patients with murine typhus as was noted earlier in patients with epidemic typhus. In a similar manner the Weil-Felix reaction in murine typhus is essentially identical with that in epidemic typhus.

On the basis of such evidence as has been presented in Figs. 2 and 3, it may be concluded that when the complement-fixation or the agglutination reaction is employed with proper antigens, it is possible to differentiate between epidemic and murine typhus. The results so far discussed are those obtained in patients exposed to the antigens of epidemic or murine typhus for the first time. A somewhat different response is obtained in persons who have been previously vaccinated with epidemic typhus vaccine and who subsequently develop infection with either R. prowazeki or R. mooseri. During World War II several million military personnel were immunized against epidemic typhus. Only a few of these many persons developed epidemic typhus during exposure to the disease in various theaters of combat; as a matter of fact, only some sixty-odd cases occurred in the entire Army during the war. In these individuals the serological response was similar to that obtained in unvaccinated persons who developed this disease. The only notable differences were that specific complement-fixing and agglutinating antibodies appeared earlier in the course of the disease and that the Weil-Felix reaction generally was of little consequence.

Persons who have been immunized against epidemic typhus and who at a later date contract murine typhus (for the epidemic vaccine does not protect against murine typhus) develop a peculiar antibody pattern. This was first demonstrated by Plotz and Wertman (9) at the Army Medical School. Fig. 4 presents the data on the original twelve cases reported by these workers plus eighteen cases collected since their report (10). The method of graphing employed here is somewhat different from that used in previous figures; the average titers obtained with sera collected from the group in certain periods of the disease are given. The solid columns represent the values as determined with epidemic antigen, and the hatched columns, the titers with murine antigen. These individuals showed higher complement-fixing antibody titers when tested with epidemic antigen than they did when tested with murine; this was true throughout the period of observation.

The values obtained when the same antigens were used with the same sera in the agglutination test gave different results (10). Here, as is illustrated in Fig. 5, the titers with murine antigen were consistently higher than those with epidemic antigen. Thus, in this group

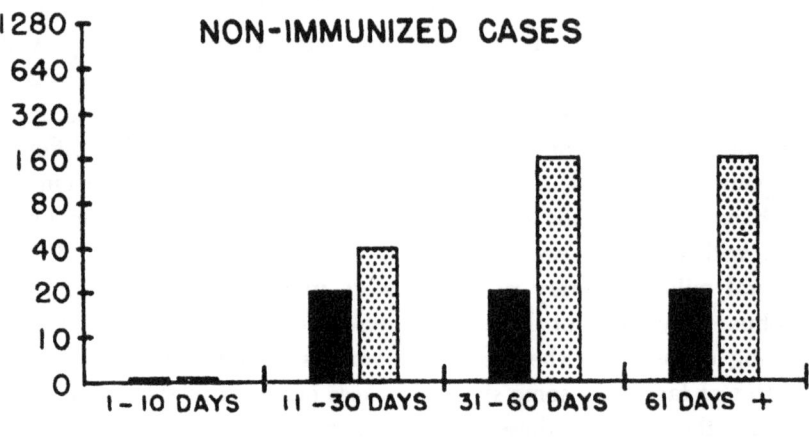

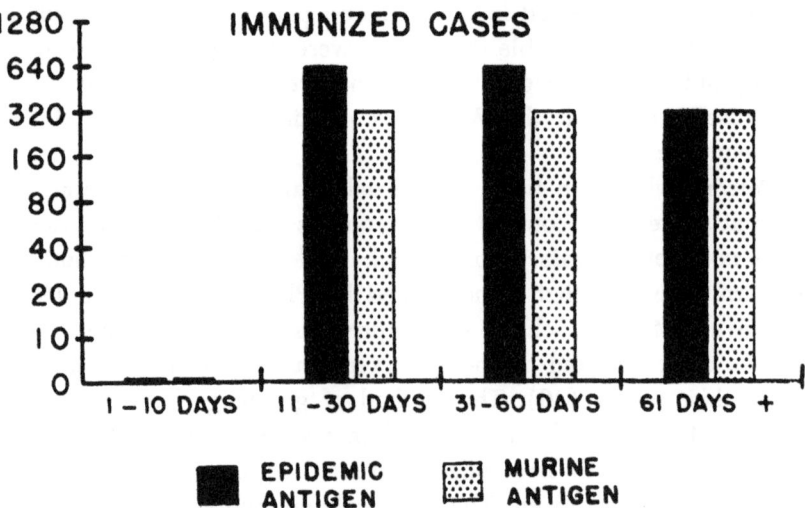

FIGURE 4. COMPLEMENT FIXING ANTIBODIES IN CASES OF MURINE TYPHUS FEVER WITH AND WITHOUT VACCINATION FOR EPIDEMIC TYPHUS FEVER
From Feldman (10)

of cases the complement-fixation reaction did not provide data which would enable the physician to diagnose properly the type of infection. Indeed, if the complement-fixation test alone were used for these cases,

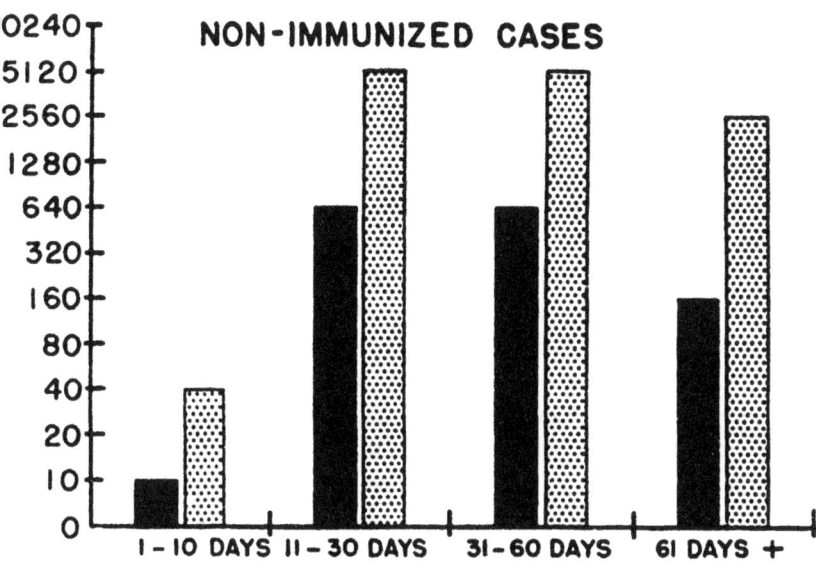
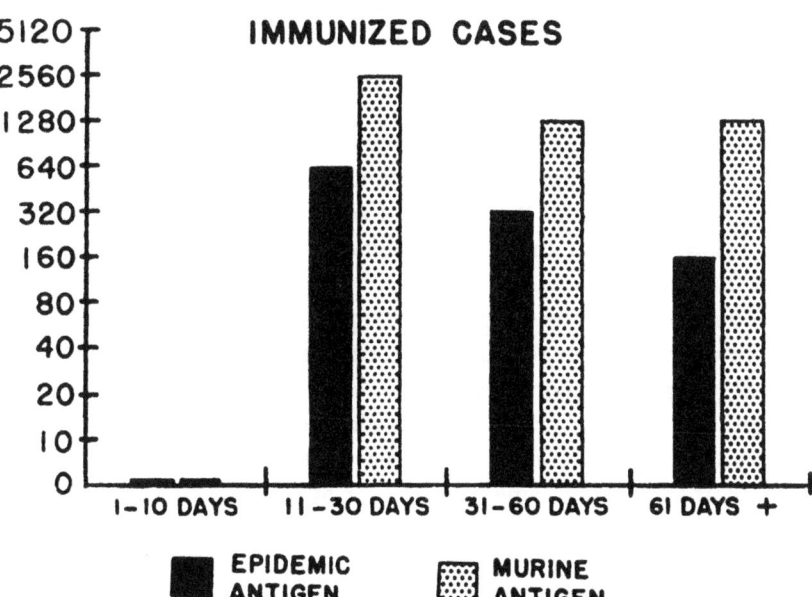

FIGURE 5. RICKETTSIAL AGGLUTININS IN CASES OF MURINE TYPHUS FEVER WITH AND WITHOUT VACCINATION FOR EPIDEMIC TYPHUS FEVER
From Feldman (10)

the interpretation might erroneously have been epidemic typhus. Fortunately, with this group of cases the agglutination reaction gave appropriate diagnostic data. It is generally assumed that this peculiar response is dependent upon an anamnestic type of reaction. It will be recalled that the soluble antigen is common to epidemic and murine typhus and that these individuals had received an antigenic stimulation with epidemic vaccine containing both rickettsiae and soluble antigen. Presumably, on becoming infected with the murine organism, the patients remembered their previous response to the common typhus antigen and promptly developed antibodies against it. Just why it is possible to differentiate between the two types of infection by means of the agglutination reaction remains to be determined.

You might wonder why I have spent so much time with this group of cases, which makes up a small proportion of patients who have been studied by various workers in the last few years. But not only is this group important from the academic point of view in immunology, it is of considerable practical importance to you in the practice of medicine during the next few years. Several million men were immunized with typhus vaccine during World War II. Presumably, for some time to come, if these persons contract murine typhus, they will respond as did the group under discussion. Therefore, it is important that you obtain a history of vaccination against typhus. Many veterans may not recall whether they received such vaccine; but, if they served overseas with any of the military units, it is safe to assume that they were immunized.

To summarize: The diagnosis of epidemic and murine typhus is largely dependent on serological procedures. The Weil-Felix reaction is still of great importance in the early presumptive diagnosis of typhus. The final laboratory data which confirm the diagnosis of typhus and which differentiate between the type of infecting rickettsiae are obtained by complement-fixation or agglutination tests employing highly specific antigens. I have said little about the relatively crude rickettsial antigens which were used until recently. These contain the specific components of either epidemic or murine rickettsiae, but, in addition, they contain the antigens common to both organisms. Therefore, with them it is difficult or impossible to differentiate between the types of infecting rickettsiae. It is my opinion that data obtained with such group-reacting antigens are of no more value than the data obtained from the Weil-Felix test. If rickettsial antigens are to be employed, then the best available antigens should be used, that is, the washed highly type-specific antigens, since here in New York City you may encounter both epidemic typhus in the form of Brill's disease among immigrants from eastern Europe, and murine typhus acquired from infected fleas of rats.

The diagnosis of Q fever by serological means is highly satisfactory and is recommended for general use. Specific complement-fixing antibodies which react with R. burneti appear toward the end of the second week and increase to a maximum during the fourth week. There are few, if any, individuals who fail to develop complement-fixing antibodies following infection with Q fever. This was demonstrated particularly in the work of the group at the 15th Medical General Laboratory, who studied the outbreaks of Q fever among our troops in the Mediterranean Theater during the latter days of World War II (11). It is of interest that the first of the modern rickettsial complement-fixing antigens prepared from infected yolk sacs for use in the diagnosis of human disease was that of Q fever. While some modifications have been made in the method since Bengtson (12) originally employed it in 1941, the principles remain essentially the same.

Certain workers prefer the rickettsial agglutination technique for the diagnosis of Q fever. However, when this method is used, the antibody response is not regularly demonstrated until some time after the complement-fixation test has become positive, the titers are generally lower, and more antigen is required for the test.

Various strains of R. burneti recovered in different geographic areas appear to be closely related but not identical. Thus, all strains are indistinguishable in cross-immunity tests in animals, and each strain elicits the same type of antibody response in human beings or in animals; nevertheless, the complement-fixing antigens prepared from different organisms vary somewhat (13). This difference is clearly illustrated in Fig. 6. Here are summarized the serological responses of guinea pigs following immunization with vaccines prepared from the Henzerling (Italian) strain and the Dyer (American) strain of R. burneti (14). Samples of blood taken at frequent intervals were tested with complement-fixing antigens prepared from both strains. It is apparent that irrespective of the type of vaccine administered, the

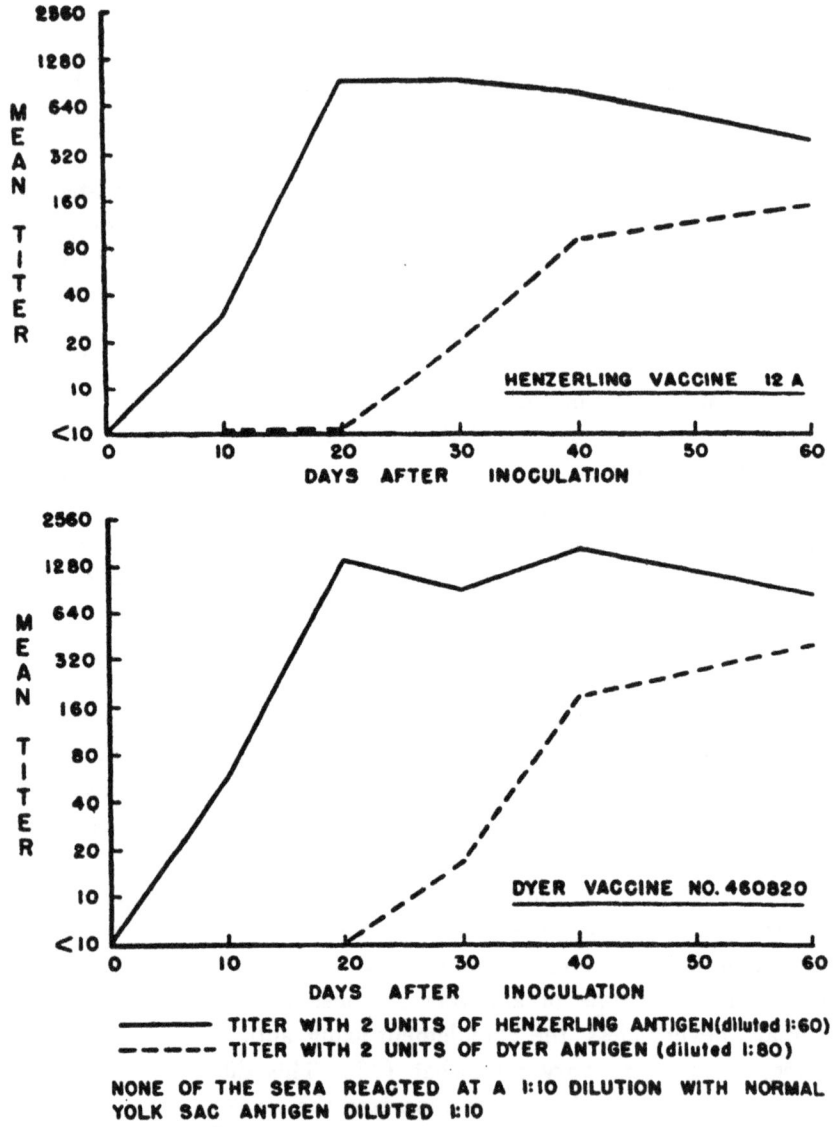

FIGURE 6. DEVELOPMENT OF SPECIFIC COMPLEMENT FIXING ANTIBODIES IN Q FEVER VACCINATED GUINEA PIGS
From Smadel et al. (14)

animals developed antibodies detectable with the Henzerling antigen on about the tenth day; furthermore, that these increased until about the twenty-first day. The titers given here are average titers for groups of about a dozen guinea pigs each; the variations of individual pigs from the average were minor. In contrast, antibody detectable with the Dyer antigen did not appear until after about three weeks and then gradually increased until the sixtieth day, at which time the antibody titers determined by the two antigens were essentially identical.

The difference in serological pattern displayed by human beings when their blood is tested with the Henzerling and Dyer antigens is even more striking. Sera from very few patients, when tested with Dyer antigen, show detectable complement-fixing antibodies even after two or three months. On the other hand, they regularly develop antibodies toward the end of the second week when the Henzerling antigen is employed. For this reason it is the practice at the Army Medical Department Research and Graduate School to use only antigens prepared from the Henzerling strain in the serological diagnosis of disease in human beings suspected of having Q fever.

No cases of naturally occurring Q fever have been reported in New York City or its vicinity. However, until 1946 only one or two cases of naturally acquired Q fever were described in the entire United States. Following the impetus to the study of this disease given by the outbreaks among military personnel in the Mediterranean Theater, a number of sharp, localized outbreaks of Q fever have been recognized in the United States. These have occurred in Amarillo, Texas, in Chicago, Illinois, and in Los Angeles, California. The illness of most of the patients in these outbreaks was first diagnosed on clinical grounds as atypical pneumonia. The cases in the United States, like those in Australia, where the disease was first recognized and named, were associated with cattle. Two methods of infection are believed to occur in Australia and presumably in the United States. *R. Burneti* is capable of infecting a number of varieties of ticks, which then excrete viable organisms in their feces. Those ticks which feed on cattle may infect the cattle and also deposit infected feces on their hides. Slaughterhouse workers and others associated with the handling of such infected cattle may acquire the disease by inhaling the dried infected tick feces on the hides of cattle or by contact with the infected carcass. Ticks infected with Q fever have been found in Pennsylvania (Parker, cited in 11). Whether they also occur in New York State has not yet been determined, but there is little reason to suppose that such ticks respect the Pennsylvania-New York state border.

To summarize: The possibility of Q fever should be suspected in persons who have contact with cattle and who develop a febrile illness accompanied by signs of interstitial pneumonia. The organism of Q fever, *R. burneti*, is readily isolated in animals or embryonated eggs inoculated with materials from patients, but this technique is so dangerous that laboratory workers should avoid this diagnostic method. The Weil-Felix reaction with OX-19, OX-2, and OX-K is consistently negative in Q fever. The serological response, as determined by complement-fixation tests using specific Q fever antigens of the appropriate strains, is sufficiently uniform so that this method provides the best diagnostic procedure for Q fever.

The diagnosis of scrub typhus is based on a history of exposure in an area where scrub typhus is endemic. The disease is found in Asia and in lands touched by the western part of the Pacific Ocean; it does not occur in the Western Hemisphere. The demonstration of the primary lesion or eschar at the cutaneous site where the infected mite vector fed, assists in early diagnosis, as does the appearance of the rash about the fifth day of fever. The development of agglutinins against the OX-K strain of *B. proteus* during the second week provides presumptive evidence for the diagnosis of scrub typhus. A specific diagnosis of tsutsugamushi disease is made by recovering the rickettsiae from the blood of patients during the febrile phase. Specific serological tests employing rickettsial materials have not yet been developed sufficiently for use as standard diagnostic procedures (6).

In closing, I should like to make several general remarks on the diagnosis of virus and rickettsial diseases based on the experience of the Army Medical Department Research and Graduate School. (1) As physicians, think of the possibility of viral or rickettsial infection when you first see the patient rather than at the end of the illness, when you have abandoned all other diagnoses. (2) As soon as you suspect one of these diseases, take a 10 c.c. sample of whole, unclotted blood for serological diagnostic tests and send it to your local virus diagnostic laboratory for immediate testing or for storage until the convalescent blood sample is collected. (3) Collect sterile convalescent blood during the third week and get it to the laboratory. (4) Work hand in hand with your laboratory. Give your laboratory man a brief résumé of the clinical findings, including the date of onset of illness and your tentative diagnosis. Put the date and the day of disease on which the specimen was obtained on each sample submitted. (5) Finally, do not ask that isolation of the agent be attempted for routine diagnostic work. Isolation and identification of viral and rickettsial agents are still essentially research procedures and should be undertaken only as a collaborative study by the physician and the laboratory worker.

REFERENCES

1. Plotz, H., The interpretation of the Weil-Felix agglutination test in Rocky Mountain spotted fever, *J. Lab. & Clin. Med.*, 1946, 31:982.
2. Castañeda, M. R., Clinical and experimental aspects of exanthematous typhus in tropical regions of America; aids to diagnosis, *Puerto Rico J. Pub. Health & Trop. Med.*, 1942, 18:165.
3. León, A. P., Reacción de Weil-Felix tipo Kahn, *Rev. d. Inst. salub. y enferm. trop.*, 1945, 6:173.
4. León, A. P., Precipitación de sueros anti-tifo por la orina de enfermos di tifo exantemático, *Rev. d. Inst. salub. y enferm. trop.*, 1942, 3:201.
   León, A. P., and C. Cano, La Reacción de "fijación del complemento inversa" en el diagnóstico del tifo exantemático, *Rev. d. Inst. salub. y enferm. trop.*, 1945, 6:167.
5. Smorodintzeff, A. A., and R. V. Fradkina, Slide agglutination test for rapid diagnosis of pre-eruptive typhus fever, *Proc. Soc. Exp. Biol. & Med.*, 1944, 56:93.
6. Smadel, J. E., Serologic procedures for the diagnosis of rickettsial diseases (p. 311), in *Diagnostic Procedures for Virus and Rickettsial Diseases*, American Public Health Association (New York, 1948).
7. Plotz, H., B. L. Bennett, K. Wertman, M. J. Snyder, and R. L. Gauld, The serological pattern in typhus fever: I. Epidemic, *Am. J. Hyg.*, 1948, 47:150.
8. Scoville, A. B., Jr., B. L. Bennett, K. Wertman, and R. L. Gauld, The serological pattern in typhus fever: II. Murine, *Am. J. Hgy.*, 1948, 47:166.
9. Plotz, H., and K. Wertman, Modification of serological response to infection with murine typhus by previous immunization with epidemic typhus vaccine, *Proc. Soc. Exp. Biol. & Med.*, 1945, 59:248.
10. Feldman, H., Serological diagnosis of endemic typhus in epidemic-immunized individuals. Not yet published.
11. Robbins, F. C., R. L. Gauld, and F. B. Warner, Q fever in the Mediterranean area: report of its occurrence in Allied troops: II. Epidemiology, *Am. J. Hyg.*, 1946, 44:23.

12. Bengtson, I. A., Complement fixation in "Q" fever, *Proc. Soc. Exp. Biol. & Med.*, 1941, 46:665.
13. Robbins, F. C., R. Rustigian, M. J. Snyder, and J. E. Smadel, Q fever in the Mediterranean area: report of its occurrence in Allied troops: III. The etiological agent, *Am. J. Hyg.*, 1946, 44:51.
14. Smadel, J. E., M. J. Snyder, and F. C. Robbins, Vaccination against Q fever, *Am. J. Hyg.*, 1948, 47:71.

Chapter 12

THE DIAGNOSIS OF ROCKY MOUNTAIN SPOTTED FEVER AND RICKETTSIALPOX

By HERALD R. COX, *Section of Viral and Rickettsial Research, Lederle Laboratories Division, American Cyanamid Company*

ROCKY MOUNTAIN SPOTTED FEVER

ROCKY MOUNTAIN SPOTTED FEVER is an acute, endemic, infectious, febrile disease belonging to the spotted-fever group of diseases, which includes other identical or related diseases, such as boutonneuse fever of the Mediterranean region, Brazilian spotted fever, Tobia fever of Colombia, Choix, or pinta, fever of Mexico, Kenya fever, South African tick-bite fever, rickettsialpox, North Queensland tick typhus, and some of the tick-borne rickettsioses of Russia and India.

The causative agent of Rocky Mountain spotted fever is *Dermacentroxenus rickettsi*, Wolbach, 1919 (*Rickettsia rickettsi*, Brumpt, 1927; *R. brasiliensis*, Monteiro, 1931; *R. typhi* do Amaral and Monteiro, 1932). The only known means of transmission to animals or to man is by infected ticks.

Epidemiology. Until 1930 spotted fever was thought to be confined to the northwest mountainous sections of the United States, although a case had been reported in Indiana in 1925. At present the disease is reported from forty-three states, the exceptions being Maine, Vermont, Rhode Island, Connecticut, and Michigan. It has also been recognized in Canada (British Columbia, Alberta, and Saskatchewan) and in parts of western and central Mexico. In South America it is known to exist in Brazil (States of São Paulo, Rio de Janeiro, and Minas Geraes), in Colombia (in Cundinamarca and Santander del Sur), and possibly in Venezuela. In Brazil the disease has been called exanthematic typhus of São Paulo, or Minas Geraes typhus, whereas in Colombia it was originally designated as Tobia fever. In the United States an average of 480 cases is reported yearly (1939–46); in Brazil 663 spotted-fever cases were reported for the period 1929–42 (1), and in Canada only 12 cases were recorded between 1919 and 1939 (2).

In the western United States the greatest number of cases are reported in April and May, the season of prevalence of *D. andersoni*. In sections of higher altitudes, such as Wyoming and Colorado, the danger period may extend further into the summer. Occasional cases have been reported during the late summer, fall, and even winter months. In the eastern United States most cases occur during the summer, the season of greatest activity of *D. variabilis*.

The virulence of the infection varies with the locality and is correlated in any selected area with the maximal level of virulence of the virus strain in the local tick population. In the Bitter Root Valley of Montana the death rate for nonvaccinated adults averages about 80 percent and for children about 37.5 percent. A high case fatality rate also prevails in other parts of western Montana, in certain areas of Wyoming and Oregon, in all affected portions of northern Idaho, and along the extreme eastern edge of Washington. In other areas of the West the case fatality rate varies, with a minimum of at least 10 percent (3). On the average, however, spotted fever in the East is just about as fatal as it is in the West. In comparing data for a ten-year period (1930-39 inclusive) Topping (4) reported that the crude fatality rate for Idaho and Montana was 28.1 percent and for Maryland and Virginia, 18.4 percent. Little difference was found in the fatality rates when the two areas were compared on the basis of age. In the western states one-half of the cases (50.2 percent) occurred in persons aged forty years or over; in the eastern states this was practically reversed, the largest number (46.8 percent) occurring in persons under fifteen years of age.

Extensive bionomic studies have been confined almost exclusively to *D. andersoni*, but the following short outline of the distribution of known vectors and of those shown experimentally capable of transmitting spotted fever will serve to indicate the wide dispersal of such species and the threat they represent to man (5).

Ticks found infected in nature: In the United States—*Dermacentor andersoni, D. variabilis, Amblyomma americanum, Haemaphysalis leporis-palustris, Ixodes dentatus, Rhipicephalus sanguineus*; in Brazil—*A. cajennense, A. striatum, A. ovale, A. brasiliensis* (also *Cimex rotundatus, C. lectularius*); in Colombia—*A. cajennense*; in Mexico—*R. sanguineus, A. cajennense*; in Canada—*D. andersoni*.

Ticks shown experimentally capable of transmission: In the United

States—*A. cajennense, A. striatum, D. occidentalis, D. parumapertus marginatus, D. albipictus, Ornithodoros parkeri, O. hermsi, O. nicollei, O. turicata, O. rudis*; in Colombia—*Otocentor nitens, Ornithodoros rudis, O. parkeri, O. turicata, D. andersoni.*

Clinical picture. In many of its general aspects Rocky Mountain spotted fever resembles typhus, the chief differential points being the duration of fever and the time of appearance and location of the rash. Attacks range from mild ambulatory and abortive forms to rapidly terminating fatal infections. In vaccinated persons and young children attacks are frequently mild and atypical.

The following description is based on the appearance of the disease as it occurs in nonvaccinated adults. The incubation period ranges from two to twelve days and averages six or seven days. The actual onset, like that of typhus, may be preceded by a few days of ill-defined symptoms—listlessness, loss of appetite, and headache. Onset is commonly abrupt, with chills, profound prostration, and a rapidly rising fever that continues to mount into the second week. Muscle and joint pains are marked, and in the more severe forms epistaxis may occur early. Remissions of 1 to 3°F. are observed in the morning temperatures. The fever terminates by rapid lysis, usually at about the end of the third week, although mild cases may become afebrile before the end of the second week.

A distinctive rash usually appears on the third or fourth day, which resembles the slight mottling seen in early measles. This fades shortly, to be followed by typical rose-red maculopapular lesions characterized by first appearing on the ankles and wrists and rapidly spreading to the legs, arms, and chest. The palms and soles, and at times even the face and scalp, become involved. The abdomen is the last and least affected. Early in the course of the disease the spots are less pronounced during the morning remissions of fever, but they become progressively more distinct each day until they are definitely petechial in all but the mildest types of infection. In severe cases the spots are confluent, deep red or purplish in color, and often necrotic. In convalescence the rash is brownish, and branny desquamation occurs over the more heavily involved areas.

There are no significant hematological changes. The white-cell count usually does not exceed 15,000 but may go as high as 30,000. Nervous manifestations are common; they include headache, restlessness, insomnia, confusion, and coma. Delirium occurs in severe cases. In fulminating cases, coma usually precedes death, which commonly occurs around the end of the second week of illness.

Convalescence is slow, even in the milder cases, and complete recovery, particularly from severe infection, may require several months and sometimes even a year or longer. Disturbances of sight, hearing, and mental acuity are not uncommon, and various symptoms associated with vascular damage may be observed. It is generally considered that persons recovered from spotted fever are more or less permanently immune.

Pathological picture. The distinctive gross features are those related to the distribution and character of the cutaneous and subcutaneous lesions of the blood vessels. The extensive hemorrhages in the scrotal tissues, often with necrosis and similar lesions of the testes and their appendages, are the most characteristic gross findings in man. The spleen is always enlarged to several times the normal size, and is firm in consistency. The microscopic lesions are practically limited to the peripheral blood vessels, including those of the external genitalia. In the beginning the proliferative lesion is apparent in the vascular endothelium. Polymorphonuclear leucocytes may or may not play a part in the lesions, depending upon the degree of intensity of the reaction, before thrombosis occurs. After thrombosis, polymorphonuclear leucocytes are necessarily present. The degenerative changes found in the endothelial cells and in the smooth muscle cells of the media indicate a direct injury caused by the rickettsiae. The general reaction to the infection is shown by endothelial cell accumulation in the blood vessels of the lung, liver, spleen, and lymph nodes. The pathology of spotted-fever cases in the Rocky Mountain area and the eastern United States is essentially the same (6).

Experimental infection. Of the common laboratory animals, the guinea pig is the most suitable for experimental purposes. After inoculation of blood from human cases, the temperature usually does not rise until three or more days have passed, and generally a few passages in guinea pigs are required before the incubation period becomes fixed at two to three days. The febrile period lasts from five to fourteen days. Death, which usually occurs with well-established strains on the sixth to the eighth day of fever, is preceded by a sudden drop in temperature to subnormal. If the guinea pigs recover, the temperature begins to drop at the end of seven or eight days, and gradually reaches normal in a period of three to six days. The first visible sign of disease in male guinea pigs is swelling and reddening of the scrotal skin on the third or fourth day of fever. At this time the animal shows signs of discomfort, loss of appetite, and roughening of the coat. The scrotal reaction may develop into a necrotic condition, followed by sloughing and subsequent healing with scar formation. Necrosis and sloughing of the foot pads and ears also occur frequently.

Etiological agent. According to Wolbach (7), the distribution and morphology of *D. rickettsi* in mammalian tissues are identical in man, monkey, rabbit, and guinea pig. In tissue sections the rickettsia has the form of a minute paired organism, often surrounded by a very narrow but definite clear zone, or halo, as if encapsulated. Often the distal ends of the pairs appear to be tapered, so that they resemble minute pneumococci. The rickettsiae average about 1 micron long and from 0.2 to 0.3 micron wide. They are best stained by special methods. With Giemsa the rickettsiae take a purplish tinge; with the Castañeda method they take a light blue appearance; with the Macchiavello method they stain red. Like other rickettsiae, *D. rickettsi* is gram negative. All attempts to cultivate *D. rickettsi* on artificial media have been unsuccessful, but they grow readily in tissue cultures and in the yolk sac and the amniotic sac of the developing chick embryo.

Spotted-fever rickettsiae do not pass Berkefeld V, N, or W candles, nor Seitz S1 filter pads. They are killed in a few minutes by exposure to moist heat at 50°C., or to chemical agents, and in a few hours by desiccation at room temperature. Red and white blood cells from infected guinea-pig blood retain their infectivity even after repeated washings. At room temperature guinea-pig blood retains its infectivity for only about a week, but in the cold room it remains infectious for about two weeks. Infected guinea-pig brain and spleen suspended in glycerin, stored in sealed containers in a dry-ice box, remain infectious for periods ranging up to a year.

Diagnosis. In spite of the commonly expressed opinion that spotted fever is an easily recognized infection, errors in diagnosis may be made even by those familiar with the disease. Often it is not possible to diagnose clinically the very mild infections or the fulminating types. Furthermore, in areas where both spotted fever and murine (endemic) typhus are prevalent, an additional difficulty is encountered because of their clinical similarity.

The laboratory tests ordinarily used for diagnosis are the infection test, the Weil-Felix reaction, the protection, or virus-neutralization, test, and the complement-fixation test. In the infection test male guinea pigs are inoculated intraperitoneally with blood from the suspected case. Clotted blood, plasma, serum, or preferably whole citrated blood without preservative may be used. Once the disease is established, it may be maintained by injecting other guinea pigs intraperitoneally with the guinea-pig blood, spleen, or testicular washings taken on the second or third day of fever. By establishing the disease in guinea pigs, it is possible to apply cross-immunity tests with known strains of spotted fever or other suspected infectious agents.

The Weil-Felix test, that is, testing the patient's serum for agglutinins against various strains of proteus OX organisms, aids in limiting the probable diagnosis to the rickettsial group of diseases, but it is of no aid in differentiating spotted fever from typhus. In checking the Weil-Felix reaction, it is essential that at least two blood samples be tested, one taken as soon as spotted fever is suspected and the other between the twelfth and the fifteenth day after onset. The first sample is seldom diagnostic and is valuable chiefly as a reference point in determining whether there is a subsequent rise in titer. A titer of less than 1:320 cannot be considered definitely diagnostic. In the majority of positive serums the agglutinins for proteus OX-19 are highest in titer, but occasionally (particularly with serums from certain areas in Wyoming [3]) those for proteus OX-2 are highest. The proteus agglutinins usually appear toward the end of the second week of the disease; but occasionally they do not appear until early convalescence, and in some cases none are produced.

According to Parker (3), the protection, or virus-neutralization, test is nearly always of diagnostic value. As performed in his laboratory, duplicate mixtures are prepared, each containing 0.5 c.c. of serum and 0.1, 0.25, and 0.5 c.c. of serum-virus, respectively. The mixtures are held at room temperature for thirty minutes and then injected intraperitoneally into guinea pigs. Control animals receive the same amount of virus and normal serum. The most consistent results (neutralization of virus) are obtained with blood samples taken in convalescence, although some serums taken during lysis show definite neutralizing capacity. The neutralization test is of greater value than the agglutination test in testing blood specimens from relatively mild cases and may give even better results than the infection test.

The complement-fixation test is an additional laboratory aid and has the distinct advantage over the Weil-Felix test in that it is much more specific and may be used to differentiate spotted fever from infections of other rickettsial groups, such as the typhus, Q fever, and scrub-typhus groups. Satisfactory antigens may be prepared from rickettsiae cultivated by the agar tissue culture method of Zinsser, Fitzpatrick, and Wei (8), or by the yolk-sac method of Cox (9). The rickettsiae of the spotted-fever group, such as Rocky Mountain spotted fever and boutonneuse fever, contain soluble antigens which are released when infected yolk-sac suspensions are extracted with ether or a number of other organic solvents (10). The soluble antigen preparations are specific for the spotted-fever group and serve to differentiate this group of diseases from the typhus, Q fever, and scrub-typhus groups; but they show so much cross fixation that they cannot be used to differentiate between diseases within the group. However, Plotz, Reagan, and Wertman (11) showed that the soluble antigens responsible for cross fixation may be removed by subjecting the formolized rickettsiae to repeated centrifugation washings and that the resulting rickettsiae provide highly specific antigens, thus making it possible to differentiate between such closely related organisms as spotted fever and boutonneuse fever. It should be noted, however, that washed rickettsial body antigens, particularly those of the spotted-fever group, are very expensive to prepare, and their cost would prohibit their use in routine tests. Recently van der Scheer, Bohnel, and Cox (12) reported the preparation of purified soluble antigens from spotted-fever rickettsiae by the use of benzene extraction followed by sodium-sulfate precipitation. These antigens show group specificity only, but they possess the advantage of giving little or no fixation of complement in the presence of syphilitic sera.

Complement-fixing antibodies begin to appear on about the eighth to the tenth day after onset. As in the Weil-Felix test, it is desirable that at least two blood samples be tested—one taken as soon as spotted fever is suspected and the other between the tenth and the fifteenth day after onset. The first sample is seldom diagnostic and is of value chiefly as a reference point to determine whether a rise in titer has occurred. A titer of less than 4+ in the 1:8 dilution cannot be considered as definitely diagnostic. Complement-fixing antibodies may persist in significant titers for ten years or more after illness, whereas the Weil-Felix test becomes negative in less than a year following infection.

In our laboratory complement-fixation tests are carried out by a modified Kolmer and Boerner technique, in which overnight fixation in the icebox is used, since this method is a somewhat more sensitive one than that originally employed by Bengtson (13, 14). All antigens are titrated for hemolytic, anticomplementary, and antigenic activity. In titrating the antigens the unit of complement is determined by one-hour preincubation of the complement at 37°C. in the presence of saline solution only.

For testing immune sera, complement is titrated in the presence of two units of antigen. Complement diluted 1:30 is added to a series of tubes beginning with 0.1 c.c. and increasing by 0.025 c.c. (thus: 0.1 c.c., 0.125 c.c., 0.15 c.c., 0.175 c.c., and so forth). Sufficient saline is then added to bring the volume in each tube to 0.75 c.c. After this, 0.25 c.c. of antigen, containing two units, is added to each tube, whereupon they are incubated for one hour at 37° C. in a waterbath. Then the hemolytic system—0.25 c.c. of amboceptor containing two units and 0.25 c.c. of a 2 percent suspension of sheep red cells—is added, and the tubes are reincubated for one hour at 37°C. The least amount of complement which causes complete hemolysis at the end of the incubation period constitutes one *exact* unit.

In the test proper, twofold dilutions of serum are made in saline of which 0.25 c.c. are used per tube; 0.25 c.c. of the diluted antigen and 0.5 c.c. of complement containing two *exact* units are added. Controls of serum, antigen, red cells, and the hemolytic system are included. The mixture is incubated overnight in the chillroom. The following morning amboceptor and red cells are added, and the tests are reincubated at 37°C. for one-half hour or until the control tubes are clear.

RICKETTSIALPOX

Rickettsialpox is the name given by Huebner, Stamps, and Armstrong (15) to a newly recognized disease first reported in New York City and described independently by Sussmann (16), Shankman (17), and Greenberg, Pellitteri, Klein, and Huebner (18). It is a mild disease of rickettsial origin, characterized frequently by an initial lesion at the site of mite bite.

Epidemiology. The disease was first recognized in the Borough of Queens, New York City (17), but it is believed that the disease occurred and was listed among febrile conditions of unknown etiology for a number of years previously. According to a recent communication from Dr. Morris Greenberg, a total of at least 332 cases have been reported up to date (January 19, 1948), all from four boroughs in New York City—Bronx, Manhattan, Kings, and Queens. There were 177 cases in 1946, with 127 in the Queens epidemic area; 154 cases in 1947, again with 17 in the Queens epidemic area; and 1 case in 1948. The recovery of at least six rickettsial strains from the tissues of *Allodermanyssus sanguineus,* an ectoparasite of house mice (*Mus musculus*), indicates that human infection is acquired by the bite of mites.

Clinical picture. The disease is characterized by an abrupt onset of chills, fever, sweats, and backache, followed three or four days later by a rash. About a week prior to the onset of fever, a firm red papule appears at the site of mite bite that develops into a deep-seated vesicle, which ultimately shrinks and dries to form a black eschar. The initial lesions, found chiefly on the covered parts of the body, although they may occur on the neck, face, arms, and the dorsum of hands, persist approximately three or four weeks. In fully developed state they frequently resemble certain stages of the vaccinia vesicle. The regional lymph nodes usually become enlarged and are tender to the touch. Fever with morning remissions is often low grade at onset but usually rises rapidly to reach 103° to 104°F. and persists for about a week. The temperature gradually returns to normal by defervescence. Chills, or chilly sensations, lasting for a day or so, frequently precede the fever. Severe headache with frontal and retroorbital pains occurs in practically all cases. Backache and general muscular soreness are common early in the course of the disease, lassitude is always present, and photophobia is a not infrequent symptom. Rash apparently appears in all cases and is noticed most commonly at the onset of fever, or one or two days later. At first the lesions are maculopapular, discrete, and erythematous, but after a day or so vesicles develop in the summit of the papules. They dry to form black crusts, which ultimately fall off without producing scars. The rash may be scanty, moderate, or abundant. There is no pattern in its distribution; it may appear first on the arms, legs, abdomen, back, face, or chest. It has not been observed on the palms or soles. The duration of the rash varies from two to three days in mild cases, to ten days in the most severe. Except for fever and rash there are no unusual signs. An enlarged spleen occurs in a few cases. General lymphadenopathy is uncommon. Red blood cell counts and hemoglobin are normal. There is a moderate leucopenia, with white cells varying between 2,400 and 7,500 per cubic millimeter. The leucopenia usually lasts only during the acute illness, and the white-cell count returns to normal in about two weeks after onset of fever. Thus far apparently all patients have recovered without sequelae.

Pathology. Since there have been no deaths, the pathology in man is unknown. Recently Hershberger and Huebner (19) have reported on the histopathology of the lesions present in the skin during the course of the disease.

In mice, intraperitoneal inoculation results in definite objective signs of illness, but few deaths occur. Mice that die or that are sacrificed when moribund show a small amount of blood-tinged peritoneal fluid, enlarged lymph nodes, an enlarged, edematous liver, and a dark, engorged spleen eight to ten times its normal size. The respiratory and intestinal tracts show no gross changes. Guinea pigs inoculated intraperitoneally with tunica washings or infected yolk sac tissue show redness and swelling of the scrotum and adherence of the testes to the tunica vaginalis, which is thickened and markedly injected; moderately enlarged spleen and lymph nodes; occasional small areas of pneumonic consolidation; and frequently, indurated cutaneous and subcutaneous nodules at the site of inoculation.

Experimental infection. Wild house mice (*Mus musculus*) trapped in nonendemic areas, guinea pigs, chick embryos, and albino mice are susceptible to infection. Mice inoculated intraperitoneally show ruffled fur as early as the sixth day after inoculation. The peak of the disease is reached between the ninth and the thirteenth day, and deaths may occur at any time during this period. Both brain and spleen tissue may be used for transfer. Guinea pigs inoculated intraperitoneally with tunica washings first show a scrotal reaction about the fifth day. Onset of fever may occur from the fourth to the sixth

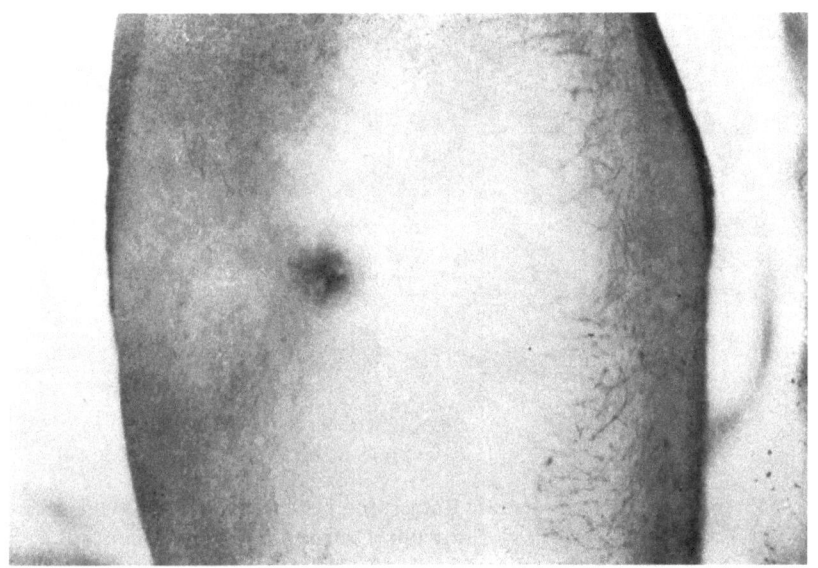

FIGURE 1. CASE OF RICKETTSIALPOX SHOWING PRIMARY LESIONS ON THE ARM

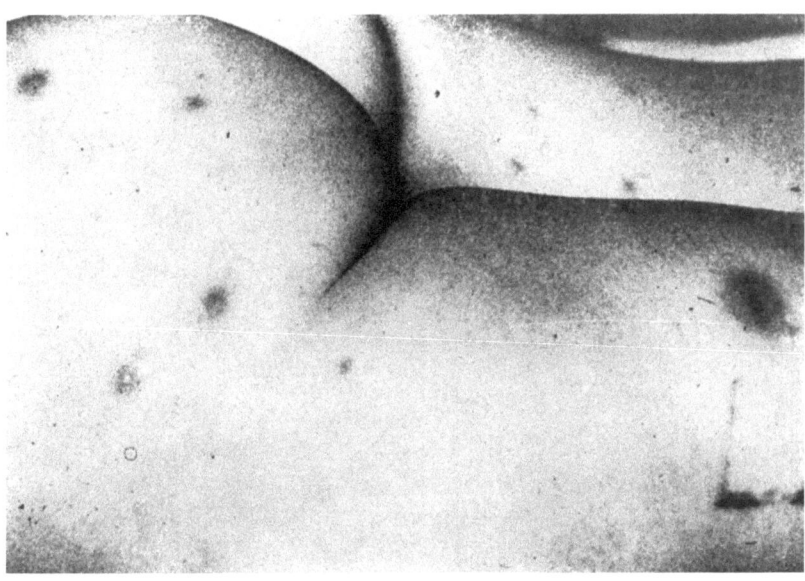

FIGURE 2. CASE OF RICKETTSIALPOX SHOWING PRIMARY LESION ON LEG AND SECONDARY LESIONS (AT RIGHT) ON LEGS AND BUTTOCKS

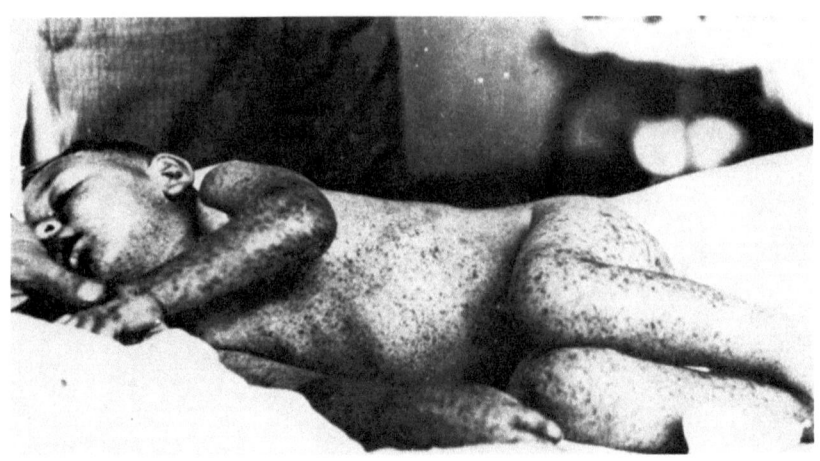

FIGURE 3. CASE OF FATAL ROCKY MOUNTAIN SPOTTED FEVER IN A FOUR-YEAR-OLD BOY, SHOWING EXTENSIVE HEMORRHAGIC RASH OVER THE ENTIRE BODY

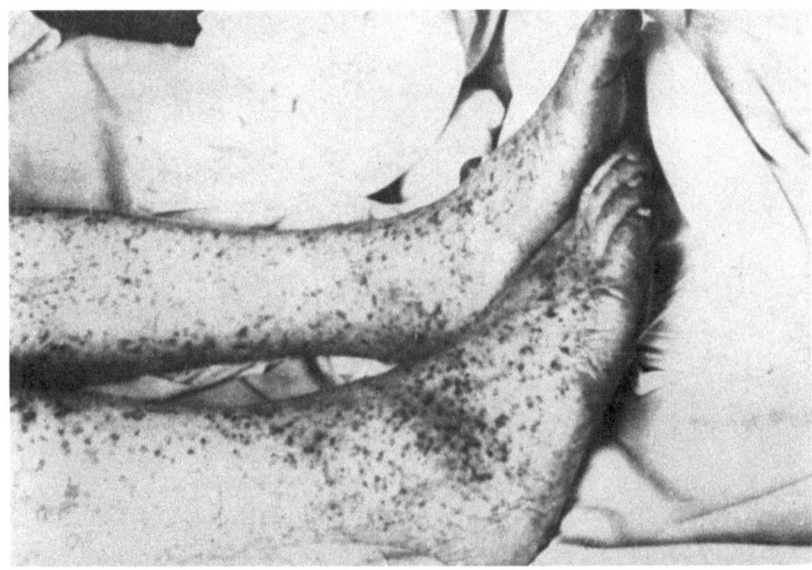

FIGURE 4. CASE OF ROCKY MOUNTAIN SPOTTED FEVER SHOWING HEMORRHAGIC RASH ON FEET AND LEGS

day. A febrile period, marked by remission, lasts for three to five days. Guinea-pig blood is not so infectious as tunica washings and gives less consistent results on inoculation. Chick embryos are highly susceptible to infection and show large numbers of rickettsiae both in the yolk sac (15) and in the amniotic sac (20). Our studies to date indicate that rickettsiae of the spotted-fever group show much better growth in the amniotic sac than do rickettsiae of the typhus, scrub-typhus, and Q fever groups. Infected yolk-sac tissue diluted 1:10 to 1:10,000 produces death of embryos in four to seven days. Guinea pigs inoculated intraperitoneally with 10 percent yolk-sac suspensions show a shortened incubation period (one to two days), followed by a sudden onset of high fever (41°C. or higher), which is sustained without remissions for four to five days. The scrotal reaction is usually delayed until the fourth day. Attempts to produce the disease in monkeys, even with massive doses of yolk-sac suspensions, have failed thus far.

Etiological agent. The etiological agent has been classified with the rickettsiae, and the name *Rickettsia akari* (GREEK, mite) has been proposed. The organism stains poorly with methylene blue and by Gram's method, but stains well with Giemsa or by Macchiavello's method. Morphologically, the red-staining diplobacillary and diplococcal forms closely resemble *R. prowazeki* and *R. mooseri*. Rickettsiae apparently are located within the nuclei of infected yolk-sac cells; in this they show properties in common with the spotted-fever group. Occasional rickettsiae are found in the peritoneum and tunica tissues of infected guinea pigs. Thus far at least, eight strains have been isolated from the blood of patients (two by Dr. Huebner and six by Dr. Rose [22]); six strains from pools of infected mites (*A. sanguineus* Hirst), which apparently is the principal vector; and one strain from a wild house mouse (*M. musculus*) trapped on the premises where cases of rickettsialpox had occurred. Available evidence indicates that the human, mite, and mouse strains are identical (23).

Diagnosis. Rickettsialpox shows many similarities to boutonneuse fever of the Mediterranean region. However, certain differences are observed. Thus, the rash in boutonneuse fever is papular or maculopapular and frequently involves the palms and soles. Monkeys are susceptible to boutonneuse fever, whereas they apparently are not susceptible to rickettsialpox. Furthermore, boutonneuse-fever, as well as spotted-fever, patients show a positive Weil-Felix reaction, whereas rickettsialpox patients apparently fail to produce agglutinins for proteus strains.

Serologically, rickettsialpox is related to the spotted-fever group in that there is cross fixation in the complement-fixation test with Rocky Mountain spotted fever. It has been our experience, with the limited number of sera at our disposal, that rickettsialpox apparently is a more sensitive antigen for certain agents in the spotted-fever group than is spotted fever; it shows not only higher titers in the presence of rickettsialpox antisera, but in many instances also with spotted-fever antisera, regardless of whether soluble or washed rickettsial body antigens are used. Thus, a satisfactory specific serological test to differentiate between spotted fever and rickettsialpox remains a problem for further study. Guinea pigs recovered from rickettsialpox show partial, but not complete, protection against spotted fever. Rickettsialpox apparently is not related serologically to murine typhus, epidemic typhus, scrub typhus, Q fever (15), or Colorado tick fever (24).[1]

REFERENCES

1. *Boletín Oficina Sanitaria Panamericana*, Las rickettsiasis en la America Latina, 1944, 23:206.
2. Gibbons, R. J., Rocky Mountain spotted fever in Canada, *Proc. Sixth Pacific Sci. Congr.*, 1942, 5:573.
3. Parker, R. R., Rocky Mountain spotted fever, *J.A.M.A.*, 1938, 110:1185, 1273.
4. Topping, N. H., Rocky Mountain spotted fever; a note on some aspects of its epidemiology, *Pub. Health Rep.*, 1941, 56:1699.
5. Steinhaus, E. A., *Insect Microbiology* (Ithaca, N. Y., 1946); Philip, C. B., Rocky Mountain spotted fever; known and potential tick vectors in the United States, *Proc. Sixth Pacific Sci. Congr.*, 1939, 5:581; Parker, R. R., C. B. Philip, and W. L. Jellison, Rocky Mountain spotted fever; potentialities of tick transmission in relation to geographic occurrence in the United States, *Am. J. Trop. Med.*, 1933, 13:341; Spencer, R. R., and R. R. Parker, Studies on Rocky Mountain spotted fever; infectivity of fasting and recently fed ticks, *Pub. Health Rep.*, 1923, 38:333; Davis, G. E., The Rocky Mountain spotted fever rickettsia in the tick genus

[1] The author is indebted to Dr. Harry M. Rose, Department of Medicine, College of Physicians and Surgeons, Columbia University, New York City, for photographs of cases shown in Figures 1 and 2, and to Dr. R. R. Parker, Director, Rocky Mountain Laboratory, Hamilton, Montana, for photographs of cases shown in Figures 3 and 4.

Ornithodoros, Proc. Sixth Pacific Sci. Congr., 1939, 5:577; The tick *Ornithodoros rudis* as a host to the rickettsiae of the spotted fevers of Colombia, Brazil and the United States, *Pub. Health Rep.,* 1943, 58:1016; Experimental transmission of the rickettsiae of the spotted fevers of Brazil, Colombia and the United States by the Argasid tick *Ornithodoros nicollei, Pub. Health Rep.,* 1943, 58:1742; Patiño-Camargo, L., Nuevas observaciones sobre un tercer foco di fiebre petequial (maculosa) en el hemisferio americano, *Bol. Ofic. Sanit. Panamericana,* 1941, 20:1112; Parker, R. R., Rocky Mountain spotted fever, *J.A.M.A.,* 1938, 110:1185, 1273; Parker, R. R., G. M. Kohls, and E. A. Steinhaus, Rocky Mountain spotted fever; spontaneous infection in the tick *Amblyomma americanum, Pub. Health Rep.,* 1943, 58:721.

6. Lillie, R. D., Pathology of Rocky Mountain spotted fever. National Instistute of Health, 1941, Bull. 177:1.
7. Wolbach, S. B., Studies on Rocky Mountain spotted fever, *J. Med. Res.,* 1919, 41:1.
8. Zinsser, H., F. K. Fitzpatrick, and R. Wei, A study of rickettsiae grown on agar tissue cultures, *J. Exp. Med.,* 1939, 69:179.
9. Cox, H. R., Use of yolk sac of developing chick embryo as medium for growing rickettsiae of Rocky Mountain spotted fever and typhus groups, *Pub. Health Rep.,* 1938, 53:2241.
10. van der Scheer, J., E. Bohnel, and H. R. Cox, Unpublished data.
11. Plotz, H., R. L. Reagan, and K. Wertman, Differentiation between fièvre boutonneuse and Rocky Mountain spotted fever by means of complement-fixation, *Proc. Soc. Exp. Biol. & Med.,* 1944, 55:173.
12. van der Scheer, J., E. Bohnel, and H. R. Cox, Diagnostic antigens for epidemic typhus, murine typhus and Rocky Mountain spotted fever, *J. Immunol.,* 1947, 56:365.
13. Bengtson, I. A., Compliment-fixation in "Q" fever, *Proc. Soc. Exp. Biol. & Med.,* 1941, 46:665.
14. Bengtson, I. A., and N. H. Topping, The specificity of the complement-fixation test in endemic typhus fever using a rickettsial antigen, *Pub. Health Rep.,* 1941, 56:1723.
15. Huebner, R. J., P. Stamps, and C. Armstrong, Rickettsialpox, a newly recognized rickettsial disease, I: Isolation of the etiological agent, *Pub. Health Rep.,* 1946, 61:1605.
16. Sussmann, L. N., Kew Gardens' spotted fever, *New York Med.,* 1946, 2(15):27.
17. Shankman, B., Report of an outbreak of endemic febrile illness, not yet identified, occurring in New York City, *New York State J. Med.,* 1946, 46:2156.
18. Greenberg, M., O. Pellitteri, I. F. Klein, and R. J. Huebner, Rickettsialpox, a newly recognized rickettsial disease, II: Clinical observations, *J.A.M.A.,* 1947, 133:901.
19. Hershberger, L. R., and R. J. Huebner, A report on the histopathology

of the cutaneous lesions of a case of rickettsialpox, *Pub. Health Rep.*, 1947, 62:1740.
20. Wong, S. C., and H. R. Cox, Unpublished data.
21. Huebner, R. J., W. L. Jellison, and C. Pomerantz, Rickettsialpox, a newly recognized rickettsial disease, IV: Isolation of a rickettsia apparently identical with the causative agent of rickettsialpox from *Allodermanyssus sanguineus*, a rodent mite, *Pub. Health Rep.*, 1946, 61:1677.
22. Rose, H. M., Personal communication.
23. Huebner, R. J., W. L. Jellison, and C. Armstrong, Rickettsialpox, a newly recognized rickettsial disease, V: Recovery of *Rickettsia akari* from a house mouse (*Mus musculus*), *Pub. Health Rep.*, 1947, 62:777.
24. Cox, H. R., Unpublished data.

Chapter 13

THE DIAGNOSIS OF INFECTIOUS HEPATITIS

By W. Paul Havens, Jr., *The Jefferson Medical College*

The concept of the viral etiology of infectious hepatitis is largely a product of investigations carried on during World War II. Actually, little is known about hepatitis virus, since it has not been successfully propagated in laboratory animals, and, up to the present, the identification of the virus rests upon its transmission to volunteers. Much of the information now available is derived from such experiments, and certain data have accumulated concerning properties of the virus and possible ways of transmission and prevention of the disease it causes (1).

At least two forms of infectious hepatitis are now recognized: (a) infectious hepatitis and (b) homologous serum jaundice. The former term, *infectious hepatitis*, is reserved for the sporadic or epidemic, naturally occurring disease. The latter term, *homologous serum jaundice*, is used to designate that form of hepatitis caused by the injection of human blood or its products containing a virus of hepatitis. Although these two forms of hepatitis are indistinguishable clinically and pathologically, certain apparent differences exist between them. These differences are concerned with length of incubation period, route of transmission, period of infectivity, location of virus in the body, and lack of cross immunity. Whether these differences indicate actually different viruses or variant forms of a single virus is, as yet, undetermined (2).

EXPERIMENTAL INFECTION AND HOST RANGE

The spontaneous appearance of hepatitis in pigs (3), mice (4, 5), and puppies (6), and its appearance in horses (7) following inoculation with homologous serum have been described. There is no evidence, as yet, that any relationship exists between the agents causing these forms of hepatitis and hepatitis in man.

Andersen and Tulinius in Denmark (3) reported that duodenal fluid obtained from patients in the acute phase of epidemic hepatitis would produce hepatitis in young pigs two to five days following ingestion. An effort was made to establish an etiological relationship between porcine and human hepatitis on the basis of experimental and epidemiological data. Limited attempts to confirm this work have been unsuccessful (8, 9).

Several attempts to transmit the virus of hepatitis to embryonating hen's eggs (10, 11) and to a variety of animals, such as guinea pigs, white mice, rabbits, hamsters, kittens, gerbils, baboons, chimpanzees (12), rhesus monkeys and other species (cercopithecus, erythrocebus, and colobus monkeys) have been unsuccessful (13). Unconfirmed reports have described the propagation of this virus in embryonating eggs (14, 15, 16) and canaries (17, 18). More recently, MacCallum and Miles (19) have reported the production of hepatitis in rats on a deficient diet, by feeding duodenal fluid from patients in the acute phase of the disease. Subsequent passage experiments in their hands failed to confirm earlier observations.

SEROLOGY

Numerous attempts to develop a specific diagnostic test for infectious hepatitis have been unsuccessful, although certain serological responses have been observed. Precipitin tests employing both acute-phase serum and cholesterolized extracts of human liver as antigens with convalescent-phase serum as antibody have been described (20, 21). Eaton et al. (22) have demonstrated an antibody in the sera of patients with acute hepatitis, which fixes complement with alcohol-soluble antigens extracted from both normal liver and liver from patients dying of hepatitis. These tests are all apparently unrelated to infectivity and have little practical value. It has also been reported that the sera of some patients with hepatitis have an heterophile antibody which is absorbable on boiled guinea pig kidney (22). In a recent survey of large military groups and carefully studied human volunteers, less than 1 percent of men had titers of heterophile antibody as high as 1:56, and this was absorbed on boiled guinea pig kidney (23).

The lack of a specific serological test and of a susceptible laboratory animal has made diagnosis dependent on the information derived from clinical and epidemiological data, in conjunction with certain tests of hepatic function.

CLINICAL COURSE OF ACUTE HEPATITIS

After onset, the clinical course of infectious hepatitis and that of homologous serum jaundice are indistinguishable. Certain differences have been evident, however, in length of incubation period and type of onset. Thus, the incubation period of the naturally occurring disease is usually twenty to forty days; in homologous serum jaundice it is longer, ranging from forty to one hundred and sixty days. The onset of disease in the former is more frequently abrupt; in the latter it is more frequently insidious.

Infectious hepatitis is said to be most common among children, in whom the course of disease is qualitatively similar, although shorter and milder than in adults. Many patients, both juvenile and adult, do not become jaundiced. If jaundice occurs, the course of disease may usually be separated into two phases—*preicteric* and *icteric*. The onset may be insidious, with anorexia, nausea, vomiting, and upper abdominal distress, or it may be abrupt, with fever, chilly sensations, and headache, in addition to the gastrointestinal complaints. Posterior cervical lymphadenopathy is frequently present. Leukopenia with relative lymphocytosis is common in the preicteric phase. Jaundice usually appears after five to seven days when the fever disappears. The liver frequently becomes enlarged and tender, and splenomegaly occasionally occurs. After the appearance of jaundice, the gastrointestinal complaints continue for one to two weeks, when jaundice reaches its height, and then regress as icterus wanes. Jaundice usually persists for three to four weeks, but it may last as long as several months. The prognosis is good in children and young adults, but the death rate may be higher in older people.

Differential diagnosis. Early in the disease, in the preicteric phase, anorexia, tenderness to percussion over the liver, and posterior cervical adenopathy may be of assistance. Palpation of the epigastrium frequently causes nausea. Evidence of dysfunction of the liver may be indicated early by certain tests. The bromsulfalein dye retention is usually the first to become abnormal, and this may occur as early as the second day of fever. The cephalin-cholesterol flocculation and then the thymol turbidity tests become positive, and ordinarily bilirubin appears in the urine at the end of the preicteric phase *before* jaundice is apparent. During the preicteric phase, leukopenia, with lymphopenia and subsequent neutropenia, is characteristic. Relative lymphocytosis, with numerous large atypical lymphocytes, appears late in the preicteric phase (24).

During the febrile preicteric phase, the diseases usually considered are: acute bacillary dysentery, typhoid and paratyphoid fever, malaria, sandfly fever, dengue, and infectious mononucleosis. The subsequent course of disease, the geographic location, and the demonstration of specific causative agents or their antibodies make the distinction evident. Of particular interest is the fact that the atypical lymphocytes found in infectious hepatitis are not to be differentiated from the cells usually considered pathognomonic of infectious mononucleosis. The presence of posterior cervical adenopathy in hepatitis and the evidence of hepatic dysfunction in a large percentage of patients with mononucleosis make differential diagnosis between them often difficult at this stage. Differentiation from acute infections of the respiratory tract may not be easy, and evidence of inflammation of the nose and throat varies in frequency with different outbreaks of infectious hepatitis. The presence of anorexia, and a sense of nausea on palpation of the epigastrium are often suggestive of the diagnosis of infectious hepatitis. Vomiting and abdominal pain with slight fever often suggest acute appendicitis. The normal or low leukocyte count and the absence of localized tenderness in the right lower quadrant of the abdomen in infectious hepatitis assist in differentiating it from appendicitis.

When jaundice is evident, the following conditions may be considered: In acute and subacute cholangitis, the leukocytosis, recurrent chills and fever, and the increased amount of serum alkaline phosphatase are helpful for differentiation from infectious hepatitis. Weil's disease may be distinguished by leukocytosis, severe muscular pain, conjunctival hemorrhages, the demonstration of the causative *Leptospira icterohemorrhagica*, and the development in convalescence of the appropriate positive serological tests. Yellow fever must be considered as a more remote possibility, depending on the geographic area and on the epidemic circumstances.

Jaundice may occasionally develop in a variety of acute and chronic infections, as in malaria, brucellosis, and amoebiasis, occasionally in pneumococcal pneumonia, general septicemias, syphilis, both congenital and acquired (secondary), and not infrequently in infectious mononucleosis. Jaundice developing during the course of malaria or amoebiasis may be differentiated by the demonstration of the respective causative parasites, while jaundice occurring during the course of infectious mononucleosis may be distinguished by the appearance, after the first week, of a characteristic course with more pronounced lymphadenopathy. Leukocytosis is common in infectious mononucleosis, and a transient and fairly high increase in heterophile antibody titer occurs often at titers of 1:128 to 1:1,024 or more. Elevated titers may also occur rarely in patients with infectious hepatitis, but they seldom reach a titer of 1:56, and the heterophile antibody in hepatitis is absorbable on guinea pig kidney.

Types of jaundice to be distinguished, in addition to those associated with various infections, include: (a) hemolytic, either congenital or acquired from various toxic agents; (b) hepatocellular, resulting from toxicity of chemicals, notably the halogenated hydrocarbons—cirrhosis of the liver; and (c) obstructive, due to extra- or intrahepatic obstruction of the biliary tract by calculus or neoplasm.

The differential diagnosis of jaundice is difficult in older patients. This is particularly true at the present time, when the occurrence of homologous serum jaundice after transfusions of plasma and/or blood is apparently increasing. Careful evaluation of the history, physical examination, and use of certain tests of hepatic function are necessary for correct diagnosis. Even with all the information available from thorough study, however, the final diagnosis, particularly in older patients, must occasionally be made by biopsy of the liver or by exploratory laparotomy.

SUMMARY

Because of the lack of a specific laboratory test and a susceptible laboratory animal, the diagnosis of infectious hepatitis depends on information derived from clinical and epidemiological data and certain tests of hepatic function. In the preicteric phase of hepatitis, differentiation from several other acute infectious diseases is frequently difficult. In the icteric phase, diagnosis may also be a problem at times, particularly in older patients. The possibility of artificial transmission of virus by the use of improperly sterilized needles used to draw blood or give injections requires emphasis. Particular attention should be directed to the history of reception of human blood or plasma at an appropriate interval (forty to one hundred and sixty days) before the appearance of icterus. The apparent increase of homologous serum jaundice in civilian hospitals at the present time frequently constitutes a difficulty in differential diagnosis of jaundice in older patients in whom the possibility of organic obstruction is great.

REFERENCES

1. Neefe, J. R., Recent advances in the knowledge of "virus hepatitis," *Medical Clinics of North America*, Philadelphia number, 1946 (Nov.): 1407.
2. Havens, W. P., Jr., The etiology of infectious hepatitis, *J.A.M.A.*, 1947, 134:653.
3. Andersen, T. T., and S. Tulinius, Etiology of hepatitis epidemica (epidemic jaundice), *Acta Med. Scandinav.*, 1938, 95:497.
4. Nicolau, S., R. Porticala, and A. Motoc, The presence of inclusions in epidemic icterogenic hepatitis (preliminary communication), *Annals Victor Babes Inst.*, 1944, 14:266.
5. Olitsky, P. K., and J. Casals, Certain affections of the liver that arise spontaneously in so-called normal stock albino mice, *Proc. Soc. Exp. Biol. & Med.*, 1945, 60:48.
6. Rubarth, S., Bidrag till den patolog-anatomiska bilden och etiologin vid den s.k. toxiska leverdystrofin hos hund, *Särtryck ur Skandinavisk Veterinartidskrift*, 1945, p. 356.
7. Slagsvold, L., Hepatitis in horses following administration of antianthrax horse serum in Norway, *Norsk. Vet. Tidskrift*, 1938, 50:69.
8. Smadel, J. E., Personal communication.
9. Ward, R., Personal communication.
10. Havens, W. P., Jr., Unpublished observations.
11. Hoyle, L., A note on some unsuccessful attempts to demonstrate a virus in infective hepatitis, *Med. Res. Council, Monthly Bull. Ministry of Health and Emergency Pub. Health Lab. Service*, 1943, 2:99.
12. Havens, W. P., Jr., and R. Ward, Failure to transmit infectious hepatitis to chimpanzees, *Proc. Soc. Exp. Biol. & Med.*, 1945, 60:102.
13. van Rooyen, C. E., and I. Gordon, Some experimental work on infective hepatitis in M. E. F., *J. Roy. Army Med. Corps*, 1942, 79:213.
14. Siede, W., and G. Meding, Zur Ätiologie der Hepatitis epidemica, *Klin. Wschr.*, 1941, 20:1065.
15. Siede, W., and K. Luz, Zur Atiologie der Hepatitis epidemica; weitere Untersuchungen zum Virusnachweis, *Klin. Wschr.*, 1943, 22:70.
16. Essen, K. W., and A. Lembke, Zur Atiologie der Hepatitis epidemica, *Med. Ztschr.*, 1944, 1:99. (Abst. in *War Med.*, 1945, 6:143.)
17. Herzberg, K., Der Kanarienvogel als Versuchstier in der Hepatitis contagiosa-forschung, *Klin. Wschr.*, 1943, 22:676.

18. Dresel, E. G., B. Meding, and E. Weineck, Uber das Virus der Hepatitis epidemica, *Ztschr. f. Immforsch. ü. exper. Therap.*, 1943, 103:129.
19. MacCallum, F. O., and J. A. R. Miles, A transmissible disease in rats inoculated with material from cases of infective hepatitis, *Lancet*, 1946, 1:3.
20. Sawyer, W. A., K. F. Meyer, M. D. Eaton, J. H. Bauer, P. Putnam, and F. F. Schwentker, Jaundice in army personnel in the western region of the United States and its relation to vaccination against yellow fever, *Am. J. Hyg.*, 1944, 40:35; *Ibid.*, 1944, 39:337.
21. Olitzki, L., and H. Bernkopf, A precipitation test in infective hepatitis, *J. Infect. Dis.*, 1945, 77:60.
22. Eaton, M. D., W. D. Murphy, and V. L. Hanford, Heterogenetic antibodies in acute hepatitis, *J. Exp. Med.*, 1944, 79:539.
23. Havens, W. P., Jr., J. M. Gambescia, and M. Knowlton, Results of heterophile antibody agglutination and Kahn tests in patients with viral hepatitis, *Proc. Soc. Exp. Biol. & Med.*, 1948, 67:437.
24. Havens, W. P., Jr., and R. E. Marck, The leukocytic response of patients with experimentally induced infectious hepatitis, *Am. J. Med. Sci.*, 1946, 212:129.

SYMPOSIA OF
THE SECTION ON MICROBIOLOGY
THE NEW YORK ACADEMY OF MEDICINE

1. DIAGNOSIS OF VIRAL AND RICKETTSIAL DISEASES
   Edited by Frank L. Horsfall, Jr.

2. EVALUATION OF CHEMOTHERAPEUTIC AGENTS
   Edited by Colin M. MacLeod

Bei Fragen zur Produktsicherheit wenden Sie sich bitte an:
If you have any questions regarding product safety,
please contact:

Walter de Gruyter GmbH
Genthiner Straße 13
10785 Berlin
productsafety@degruyterbrill.com